SOMEBODY'S GOT TO DO IT

Making History in a Big City Fire Department

by

JOHN BANKHEAD
PFD, RN, BSN (retired)

GYPSY
PUBLICATIONS

Published in 2014, by Gypsy Publications
Troy, OH 45373, U.S.A.
GypsyPublications.com

First Edition
Copyright © John Bankhead, 2014

Bankhead, John
Somebody's Got to Do It: Making History in a Big City Fire Department
/ by John Bankhead

ISBN 978-1-938768-40-8 (paperback)

Library of Congress Control Number
2014939724

Cover and Book Design by Tim Rowe

PRINTED IN THE UNITED STATES OF AMERICA

DEDICATION

This book is dedicated to the men and women of the Philadelphia Fire Department

Fr. Ronald Nyari and Anne Nyari who spent time helping me with all the things that made this book possible.

Lt Dave Schectman who at times had a better memory than me.

My beautiful wife Janet, who I couldn't live without.

Meaghan Fisher of Gypsy Publishing who made the people in my memory come back to life.

Editing by the best, Renee Manastrumi

Cover art from Tim Rowe whose work catches the essence of unrestrained danger

TABLE OF CONTENTS

PROLOGUE

The street looks different now; the fire station is long gone, burned to the ground when the lumber yard next door caught fire. The men working there when I was assigned, are all dead now, with only myself and the odd one or two left to remember the fires of long ago. The days of the wooden ladders and iron men have long passed out of memory, replaced by the modern equipment and air-pack toting men in yellow helmets. The apparatus are twice as big, driven by men in comfortable isolation from the elements. Gone is the roar of engines without mufflers, the roto lights, and the federal sirens. These are now just pictures in old books. Gone are the men riding the back step, knees bent, trying to close their coats while holding on with one hand, in the pouring rain. They dodged the bottles and bricks thrown from rooftops at the passing firemen on the way to a false alarm. The old firehouse conversations about "Harry the Match" who tried to burn down North Phillie, and almost succeeded are only a memory. I still recall the night we found him burned to death next to his gas can in the hallway of a vacant house.

Standing on the roof of a burning brownstone, watching five other fires raging on neighboring streets, these memories are all that are left. After graduating from fire training school I experienced the new man indoctrination of having to wrap up all the dead bodies, until the next class graduated from Fire School. The old timers gave every dirty, disgusting back-breaking job to the new man, until he was accepted by the others, who then shared the work. I remember how all the bullies surfaced when a new man was assigned, and the dozens of dirty tricks they thought up.

It was a chapter in the annals of the Philadelphia Fire Department that needs to be recorded, before we all are gone. All the men who slugged it out toe to toe, over kitchen arguments, but who went to bat for one another time and again in the brotherhood we all cherished. We worked on each other's homes and cars, and our wives all knew each other.   When you needed them, you were not forgotten.

After the terrible accident that made me take stock of how many brushes with death I had had, and with my family in mind, I made a decision to transfer out of Engine 2 and Ladder 3. Making the transition to Fire Rescue made me realize that I preferred to work the streets without an officer, and a pecking order of Type "A" personalities. I enjoyed being put on the spot, and preferred to trust in myself to make the right call when necessary. I came to enjoy the schooling, learning the new equipment, and work-ing with the best-trained partners dedicated to "making a difference". We handled everything that happened in the big city, packaging every patient into a nice clean accept-able bundle for the emergency rooms. How we did what we did with only two men amazed me every day, and we could not have succeeded without enlisting scores of civil-ians to assist at crucial times. We saw the spark of life drain from so many, and helped that spark to reignite in the wonderful people we snatched back from death. With time as a formidable enemy, one extra car in our path, spelled death for so many. Just that 30 seconds was all we needed to make the impossible a reality.

As a paramedic, I found that the demand for our services was so great that we were in danger of running out of gaso-line almost every shift. Many times we had to go out of service to fill the tank, or change shifts in the center lane of

Market Street with the siren blaring on the way to another call. Of my days on the job, I remembered my time in the Fire Rescue Service as the most well spent, and I'm sure that my many partners felt the same. The respect from physicians and nurses came grudgingly, until they saw the changes wrought by these interlopers into their world of medicine. The enlightenment for us came very rapidly at first, and the surprise for all of us was in how well early intervention worked. For the first several years, unfettered, we went about the business of making hearts work again, and these are the stories from that time.

The original young energetic doctors who initiated the service went on to other endeavors. The original crews were transferred out as the service expanded. Layers of supervisors were added, and the service settled into a level of service enjoyed by other big cities. The times were changing, and the service was moving on from those very first years where we followed aggressive protocols to the letter. I wouldn't be around very long to see the squads of the future; I found a lump in my groin one night at work, and embarked on the fight of my life, a battle with cancer. I was always contented with my years in the Fire Department, because I realized, "Somebody's got to do it." I was glad it was me.

THE BEGINNING OF MY CAREER IN THE PHILADELPHIA FIRE DEPARTMENT

About tem minutes into the exam, about half the room was empty, as one after the other, the men stood up and left.

I had just worked an evening shift at a pizza shop, and was fast asleep when a group of friends stopped by the house on their way to take the fire department exam. I awakened to them ringing the doorbell, and lurched out of bed to answer it. When they explained that it was the morning of the test for the Philadelphia Fire Department, I remembered that we had filled out applications months before. I had previously received a postcard allowing me to take the exam, and had put it in a drawer in my bedroom. They had completely caught me off guard, and agreed to wait while I dressed to go with them.

On the ride to the school where the exam was to be held, the four others in the car each took turns relating what they had done in preparation for the big exam. They were all trying to impress each other with their individual preparations, citing the prep books they had mastered. I was still groggy, so I just sat back and listened to their stories with my eyes half closed in the back seat of the car.

Once we arrived, I was assigned a classroom and sat down at the desk. The exam was handed out, and I filled out the answers to the test as fast as I could. The exam was a timed event, so the work had to be done quickly. About ten minutes into the exam, about half the room was empty, as one after the other, the men stood up and left. I found the questions to be extremely difficult, and I guessed the last 10 questions. Throughout the exam men continued to stand up and leave the room, until there were only about seven of us left at the exam's end. I was beginning to feel pretty stupid for not being able to finish the exam as fast as all those men who had left before me, but most of the questions were word problems requiring you to read a scenario and answer questions about it. When I left the building, I was the last to arrive back at the car; the others were all standing around waiting for me. There was a long conversation about everything they remembered about the exam, and how each question was answered. They asked me a few questions, but I couldn't help them out. I was hungry and wanted to go home. It would be some time before the results of the exam would be mailed. It was over, and I went back to tossing pizza pies in the evening after classes.

Both my father and my uncle were in the Philadelphia Fire Department. And neither was aware that I had taken the exam. I did not tell my father because he was paying for my education at Temple University where I was enrolled in the Teachers College. I was a lousy student, totally unprepared for the unregimented campus life of an inner city school. I welcomed the chance to earn a paycheck outside of throwing pizza pies all evening.

MAKING THE GRADE

I decided to drop out of college and take the appointment.

Sometime later, I received a postcard in the mail with my grade on the exam. My mark was 78.58 which earned me a

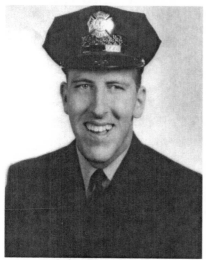

spot in the next class to be appointed in April 1962. Additional information on the postcard ranked me 82 on the list, so I decided to drop out of college and take the appointment. I checked with the friends who had taken the exam with me, and found that I was the only one to pass the Fire Department examination. To my surprise, they were very cold and somewhat annoyed to receive the

John Bankhead

information from me after admitting that they flunked the exam.

I received a notification that I had an oral exam and a physical exam to take which was accomplished in short order, then I was assigned to the fire training school. The fire training school was located in the northwest part of the city. It was a collection of buildings with an active firehouse attached. There was a fire tower and a building approximating the shape of a firehouse. The building was used to store two pieces of equipment, with classrooms on the second floor, two large garage doors in the first floor, and an adjacent tower which is five stories high. There was a net erected alongside the tower which had double windows on each floor all the way up to the roof. The net was a rope net, and it was to save any firefighters that were climbing the outside wall if they fell or dropped any of their equipment. The net was in place to catch anything before it hit the ground. The TOWER building was used for training purposes. The grounds were a large space, large enough to pull the apparatus out of the apparatus bays and conduct the various exercises that a rookie class was required to do. My initial expectation was that I would have to go through a series of physical endurance tests, like carrying a person, and moving equipment over a measured course. To my surprise, they had dreamed up a great little test of both strength and nerve. You had to climb up the outside of the fire tower using a scaling ladder. The ladder was a very heavy, awkward affair which required a good amount of strength and balance to manipulate. Like every Houdini trick, if you maintained a certain balance it was fairly easy to do, but one slip or miscalculation and you were toast. One such ladder was carried on every ladder truck; it was supposed to be used to climb the outside of a building where access could not be gained to the interior stairway. It didn't take long for me to master its use, and in several weeks we had lost some of our fear of heights. Climbing up the outside wall of a building using this ladder was unnerving for this young former student who realized that one mistake could break me like a potato chip. You had to have a lot of confidence in the ladder to swing out of a window onto it and then climb outside the building while it

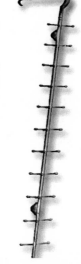

swung back and forth with every step on it. Once you got out onto the ladder, you went like a bat out of hell to climb up and get back into the window again. It's amazing what you can do with the whole class waiting on the ground looking up, wait-ing for you to make a mistake. The last thing you wanted was to err and give them a leg up on you. Drop the ladder into the net, and you would never hear the end of it; you don't get sympathy from a bunch of young Turks. It was the same as junior high school - everybody was sizing up everybody else. I had had a rough time in junior high school, and I was not going to repeat that experience here. This aspect of the train-ing was probably designed to get you to follow orders with-out engaging in the democratic process. When the officer told you to go up and get that person, you got the ladder and did what you were told without regard to your own personal safety. The risks of hanging on the outside wall of a building were secondary to completing the assignment you were ordered to do. The fruits of this labor would be realized sooner than all of us realized when a classmate was ordered to climb a ladder to retrieve a body hanging from a window, and he went up without a word. You don't realize why things are the way they are in training, until you automatically respond to something that might have been questioned if you stopped to think about it.

Another exercise that was required was to jump out of a second story window into a net held by the rest of the train-ees. This was accomplished first by a lieutenant who showed us the proper form for jumping out of the window. We went through an exercise the first day on how to hold the net, what manpower was required, and how to steer the net if the person jumped too far out from the window. This is another piece of equipment that is carried on a fire apparatus that is never used. Jumping from heights above the third floor of a building will result in severe injuries to both the jumper and the men on the net. Additionally, the time required to assemble the folded net, secure enough men to hold it, and move it to the site would probably preclude its use. Usually jumpers don't stand there thinking about it. When you are being burned you run and take a flying leap, which I have since seen.

When I got home that night, I asked my father how he

accomplished this task when he went through training. He said when it was his turn to jump from the window he just jumped into the net feet first, fell forward, and got out of the net. I decided I would do the same thing. The school however wanted you to jump out of the window and land on your backside, then they would tilt the net and you would exit the net. One of the trainees was a black fellow who appeared afraid when his turn came. He became very ill after the jump and was sent to the hospital by rescue squad. We later learned that he had a heart attack while jumping out of the window and we never saw him again. We had another trainee named Guy Bluford who only lasted a few days and he decided to go back into the Air Force, and later became an astronaut.

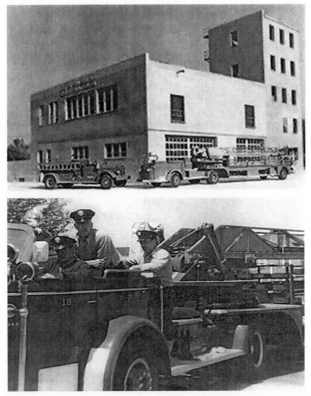

Fire Traning School 1962 & Fire Training Apparatus

BOOM

Immediately a large blue and yellow flame exited the hole and there was a loud explosion.

The class proceeded uneventfully for many weeks as I learned the basic function of fire department tools, apparatus, and how to get along in the job. During the training we were assigned to light a fire in the basement of the fire tower at the school. We poured gasoline on debris placed in the basement; then at that moment a bell rang giving us the opportunity for a break. The break lasted almost thirty minutes, during which time the liquid turned into an explosive mixture. The exercise involved throwing a lit torch down a pre-made hole in the floor to ignite the debris in the basement. After the fire had a start we were to take our hose lines and advance into the basement and first floor to put the fire out; however, we never got the chance. The source of ignition was a rag doused in gasoline placed on a long metal pole. A trainee was to advance into the first floor of the tower with the lit torch and force it down a hole in the middle of the floor which would start the fire in the basement. As he approached the hole with the lit rag on the pole he tossed it at the hole and missed. He began walking out of the room when he realized he had missed the hole with the torch, so he turned, approached the torch, and kicked it into the hole. The torch upturned and dove down towards the basement. Immediately a large blue and yellow flame exited the hole resulting in a loud explosion. All of the gasoline that had been poured into the basement turned to vapor during the break. Suddenly, everything was in disarray and all of the prepared trainees were blown backwards from their positions. I was on the hose at the doorway and found myself 20 feet away, without a helmet, facing the wrong direction. I was afraid to open my eyes because I felt a lot of stinging from things hitting my face and was afraid that items were impaled in my eyelids. I kept my eyes shut until another trainee approached me and I asked him if anything was sticking in my face and he said no. At that point I opened my eyes and discovered that all of the helmets from all of the trainees had blown from their heads and were in pieces lined up against the fence surrounding the property 30 feet away. I also discovered that the pain I had felt in my face were specks of dirt blown into my face through the open door. The basement door was blown into pieces and several are still impaled in a fire escape one story above. All of the windows in the adjacent firehouse were blown out just as several firemen were sitting down to lunch in the kitchen. Of course that activated the fire alarms in the adjacent firehouse and they brought the apparatus around to the fire training school in preparation for extinguishing the fire that started in the basement. The trainees were in no condition to go on with the exercise, since many had never experienced being in an explosion in their lives. This was my first experience with the perils of working in the Philadelphia Fire Department. Little did I realize at the time, that what had just happened to me was nothing compared to the experiences I would go through during the rest of my career. The rest of the fire school training went uneventfully and we all graduated and were assigned to companies throughout the city. It was my luck to draw one of the busiest companies in the city of Philadelphia, Engine Company 2. I did not find out until later, that my father had a hand in selecting which company I was assigned to.

A SHEEP IN WOLF'S CLOTHING

The apparatus was a big giant slug that couldn't get out of its own way, and took forever to get to a fire.

Engine 2's firehouse was located at Seventh and Norris Streets, which housed another company and a battalion chief. Also in that house were Ladder 3 and Battalion Chief 6. It was an old building and it stood in front of a very large two-story building which was the original Fire Training School that we now used as a garage. Housed on the apparatus floor were the assigned pieces of equipment, except for the chief's car which was out for repair. In place of the new car was a red 1958 Ford with a big stupid looking bell on the front. The bell was welded onto the front bumper and a rope went through the car to the seat so the chief could pull on it to ring the bell. I had the opportunity to ring it once and it went clack and didn't sound much like a bell.

The engine was a very large affair called a John Bean pumper, which supposedly put out 750 pounds of pressure at the tip of the machine gun-shaped nozzle. The gun was held in two hands, and it was used to put out small fires by using high pressure fog spray which were very small droplets of water. The small droplets are supposed to absorb the heat from the fire and extinguished the fire. There were all sorts of stories circulating among the firemen about the power the Bean pumper could put out through the gun-like tip. There were stories about the stream smashing out windows, blowing furniture over, and causing untold damage and mayhem to anything in front of it when you squeezed the trigger. It was all bullshit. The apparatus was a big giant slug that could not get out of its own way, and took forever to get to a fire. We rode on the back step, and kept looking around the sides of the apparatus hoping we could see the fire first, and get a jump on pulling the line off from either the left or right reels.

The third piece of equipment was a Maxim Magirus ladder truck. It had no tillerman seated on the back. It was a straight piece of equipment which did not articulate. Made in Germany and sold in the U.S. it featured a Nazi 88 gun mount left over from World War II, which moved the main ladder into position. It was a very ingenious design, but hard to get down small streets because it required such a large turning radius. Unlike Engine 2 it was able to put some power to the rear wheels. Being newly assigned I felt like I was a civilian in with a group of professional fire-fighters, because virtually all the training I received in fire school had no practical application in an actual firehouse. I was to start my learning all over again, and in approximately six months I had experienced most of what I would need to fulfill the rest of my time in the job. In those days firemen in an engine company would stand on the back step and hold onto a bar on the apparatus as it drove down the street. You had to keep your knees bent so when the apparatus went over a hump you would not fly up into the air. We were all instructed on the first day how to ride the apparatus. The best position was on either side of the rear step so you could look up the side of the apparatus and see where we were going. The newest man always was in the middle of the step, receiving orders from the men on the sides.

STUNNING HISTORY

I realized that all the helmets belonged to firemen from that station who had been killed in the line of duty.

It was very important when the alarm sounded in the firehouse to be the first or second guy on the apparatus. The last thing anyone wanted was to be left behind, because it was extremely serious and frowned upon if you were. I remember my first day in the firehouse, on the wall was a row of helmets and each helmet had a framed document below it. The helmets were in poor condition, they were dented and missing pieces, and as I began reading the framed information, I realized that all the helmets belonged to firemen from that station who had been killed in the line of duty. The certificate said that they were killed at an explosion at Berg Laboratories on October 28, 1954, where 12 firemen died. It seemed that the station I had been assigned to had a very active history, and many members of my station were killed in the line of duty sometimes several at a time. I didn't know what to think of it at first, so I just looked, read, and absorbed the information. I later met both officers and men on other shifts that bore large scars on their faces from fire ground injuries, caused by flying glass and pieces of metal. Being young, I had made the assumption that everything happened to someone else, and that nothing would happen to me, until I was almost killed several times in that company. I did make a mental note to have my picture taken in uniform to be posted if I was killed on the job. I always hated the high school photos in the obituary column of the paper for guys in their fifties.

Eventually an alarm came in and I was to have my first

experience at a fire. I remember riding on the apparatus thinking what the hell was I doing here. I was assigned to follow another firefighter who had graduated a couple classes before me, to follow him, and he would tell me what to do. The fire was a small affair in one room of a house. Evidently, someone had fallen asleep with a cigarette and set a chair on fire, and an adjacent table, and burned the wall. It was quickly extinguished, and I helped remove all the burned pieces of furniture and placed them on the sidewalk. There wasn't much damage to the property. It was a relatively simple fire and I got my first experience of inhaling the odors of the burnt contents in the house. It wasn't a pleasant experience, but I was intrigued by the totally unfamiliar noxious odors and smells produced by the burning contents of the home. The rest of the day passed uneventfully, and throughout the next day there were only a few short runs, several false alarms, and not much to occupy us. Little did I know what was to follow. At that time we worked two dayshifts, followed by two nightshifts, ending with two days off. Then the sequence would be repeated. On my first night work it was a summer evening and we got the call at approximately 9 to 10 o'clock at night about eight blocks away from the firehouse. This call would indoctrinate me into the full realization of what was required in the job.

OH MY GOD WHAT DID I
GET MYSELF INTO!

The body was sticking out of the window like a
flagpole with one leg trapped inside the window,
and the other draped down the wall.

As the alarm bell was ringing you could hear the pound-
ing steps of a dozen men heading for the apparatus floor.
Each was heading for his pair of boots standing upright
on the floor next to his place on the apparatus. Leaving
the station we looked toward the horizon where we could
see a reddish orange glow in the sky. Since it was dark we
couldn't see the smoke, and all that could be seen was a
distant glow as we screamed toward the location. The
closer we got, the bigger and brighter the glow looked until
eventually we could see flames licking above the rooftops.
I sensed this was going to be bad, as the men on the back
step were putting on gloves, closing up their coats, and
pulling up their boots on the way. We got to the corner
of the street where the fire was located, and the apparatus
halted briefly while I stepped backward off of it with a
length of hose in my grip. Immediately it sped off down
the street laying line as it went. I was in a race with the
pump operator to supply him water as fast as he could get
the pumper in service. As I worked on the fire hydrant, he
was connecting line to the pump. We worked as a team to
get enough water to fight the fire.

The neighborhood where the fire was located, consisted
of brick row homes, with brownstone steps on the front of
the buildings, and brownstone lintels above the windows.
These homes had been wealthy homes at one time. They

were very large, three stories high, and had since been converted to multiple occupancy apartments. The once wealthy neighborhood had now become part of a very large ghetto stretching out from the center of Philadelphia. This section was our responsibility, as our firehouse was located directly in the center of this large ghetto area. The area had a very large, poor, population the bulk of which were unemployed or unemployable.

As we proceeded into this area, what greeted us was a well-stoked fire in one of these three-story brownstone multi apartment dwellings. My first job was to stretch hose line from the rear of the pumper to a hydrant on the corner, and make the connection. The pump operator Hugh French made the connection at the other end, and put the pump into service supplying water. I had the job done in only a few minutes and as I looked up I saw flames coming from the first floor doorway and from all the windows on the first floor and all the windows on the second floor. There was a body at the second floor window level. The body was sticking out of the window like a flagpole with one leg trapped inside the window and the other leg draped down the wall. The remnants of any clothing were still burning on the body; the man was obviously dead, and his body was covered with char. We later found that his leg was trapped in a portable ladder system affixed to the base of the window. It usually had a metal cover over it, but the cover was missing. The portable ladder that was to be thrown out of the window was ajar on the floor and his foot was in the middle of it. This had firmly locked him in position with his knee at the window sill level. He was obviously standing at the window when he died, and fell forward out of the window with one leg anchored inside.

A ladder was placed on the wall adjacent to the body and Dave Schectman was ordered to go up the ladder and remove the body if possible. The neighbors were aroused, as they were screaming and yelling at the fire-fighters. There was a general uproar, and it was obvious the onlookers wanted the man removed. Dave went up the ladder took a leg lock on the rung with his leg, and grabbed the body around the waist and tried to pull it toward him. He could not accomplish his task, as the body bounced up and down but would not come loose from the window. He then asked for an axe, but Lieutenant. Jones refused fearing that the crowd would riot seeing Dave hitting him with an axe. Just then the body broke loose with a snap of the leg, and fell to the pavement. Police on the scene immediately covered the body with a disposable blanket on the pavement; however, the blanket immediately caught fire and began to burn on top of the body. A police officer grabbed the burning blanket and flung it to the rear directly over top of my head, as I was still holding the ladder. I looked up and all I saw was an orange glow of the burning blanket lying over my helmet. I reached up and tore the blanket off and threw it to the side. At that point the roof cornice gave way and tumbled down hitting Dave, narrowly missing me, showering us with burning rubble, and lacerating Dave's forearm. After Dave descended we helped load the body into the back of a police wagon. The police seemed as though they wanted out of there as soon as possible. At that point I was then ordered into the building to assist on the second floor. I went up the front steps, stepping over the puddles of aluminum on the steps from the melted storm windows and went into the building. There was a vestibule in the front burned black, and a stairway going to the second floor. To the right of the stairway was a hallway which gave access to the other rooms on the first floor of the house. Everything was black and charred and steam was coming from the walls and the floor. Water was dripping from everything, and it was extremely hot inside. There were hose lines stretching in the front door, with some going down the hallway and some going up the steps. I could hear voices and see lights on the second floor. I climbed the steps to the second floor and was directed to go to the front bedroom, the same room that had the body hanging from the window. When I got to the front room, there was already a young fellow close to my age waiting there for me, and on the floor was a pile of disposable blankets. He didn't say anything, he just pointed to what was left of a bed. There was a box spring and some metal coils that had once been the mattress. Everything in the room was burned to its framework, and had collapsed onto the floor. In the center of the bed was a body lying face down, which had integrated into the box spring and mattress springs. The initial site was very shocking because I had never seen a dead body this closely before, let alone one that had been burned as badly as this one. The spinal column bones were visible, as were the upper arm bones, elbows, heels and some bones of the skull. The entire scene was wet and glistening from water running from the ceiling while they fought the fire on the floor above. The other firefighter present asked me how I thought we were going to get that body out of the box spring. I answered him by saying, "Let's pick up the spring, turn it upside down, and shake it back and forth," which we did. Initially I had my doubts that the body would come out of the spring because it was melted so far into the center of it; however, after repeated shaking back and forth sort of like sifting sand, a heel fell down onto the floor on which we had laid a disposable blanket. As we continued to shake, another heel fell down then the entire body with a sickening thud crashed onto the floor and the real horror started. Fastened up in the center of a spring was this large, green, twisted ball of intestines with an umbilical cord type strand coming from the spring going down to the center of the body's abdomen. After repeated shaking with a sickening wet smack the rest of the intestines fell back into the body and we lay the spring back where we had found it. We wrapped up the body, placed it into a portable stretcher, (canvas with wood slats sewn in and leather handles) strapped it inside, and passed it down the stairs. We were then directed to take the remaining disposable blankets and go to a second bedroom down the hallway. In that bedroom we found a man and a woman in the bed, both dead. They were untouched by the fire, but they were black from the soot that covered everything in the room. It looked like someone had blown a dry black powder into the room freezing everything in place. The first thing I noticed was their shoes were placed side-by-side together at the foot of the bed just where they had left them. We pulled both bodies from the bed onto the floor one at a time, and wrapped each one individually, the same as we had done in the front room, and passed them down the stairs. At that time, we were directed to the rear bedroom, where again we found additional bodies. It seemed that other than the front bedroom, most of the others had their doors shut when the fire started and they all died from smoke inhalation. No one could breathe through that thick soot that had totally blanketed everything and I realized I was witnessing the aftermath of smoke inhalation. I had an opportunity to look out into the rear yard which was full of trash, old furniture, and old appliances. Piled on top of the trash were several large dead dogs which had been thrown out of the windows of the building. For some reason that I didn't understand, the fire department didn't pack up dead dogs and send them somewhere, they just threw them out the windows into the yards and that's where they lay. While we were wrapping the bodies on the second floor, it was my understanding that other firemen were packing up bodies on the third floor. I believe there were seven fatalities in this fire. Later we were informed by the police that the fire was started by an irate man who lived across the street. He was under the impression that his wife was having sex with one of the occupants in the building so he set it on fire. I didn't know which one of the bodies, if any, that I wrapped up was the offending wife, and it didn't really matter.

I couldn't believe what I had just done, having never seen a dead body before, having never touched a dead body before, and being fresh out of two years of college.

I was stunned. For some reason I thought that this was an exception rather than a rule, and it would not be repeated in my time with the fire department. Oh, how wrong I was, because time and time again the same scenario would be repeated, but in different versions of the identical scene. Initially, after the first one, I thought I would never eat bacon again, but the next morning I insisted on having bacon, because if I did not eat it, I would never eat again in my life. My impression was that the burnt bodies had looked just like bacon, and eating bacon looked just like I was eating a piece of the bodies. It was extremely distasteful, but I knew that was ridiculous. I never thought I would get used to the scenes; however, while each one carried its own shock, made its own impressions, for some reason, they never really affected me personally. As my career wound on, I had no problem dealing with adult suffering, but what really gave me a large problem and made it very difficult for me, was seeing children hurt. Every time I was deeply affected, and filled up emotionally at those sights. Hard as I was, I could never get over the sight of poor, injured children who didn't understand what had happened to them.

WHATEVER'S HANDY

*He averted his face from the attack, and received
a slicing blow down the side of his head.*

There's an area towards the front of the firehouse on
the apparatus floor where all messages are received via the
PA system; it's called the watch desk. Someone is always
present in this area to receive the alarm announcements,
and alert the company to respond. When things were slow
in the firehouse, usually, several men congregated around
this area. I was in this area one afternoon with another
fireman who was standing a two-hour watch. Through the
door came a young boy who claimed there was a problem
down the street in one of the houses which happened to
be a three-story multiple occupancy rental, with six units,
two to a floor. He said someone was injured and needed
help, so I elected to walk with him down the street, to see
what was going on. The place was typical of the houses
in our area, a large brownstone structure that had once
been a rather expensive home and now was converted to
rentals. The young boy indicated I should go up the steps
inside, because the problem was on the second floor. He
appeared to be afraid, and refused to reenter the home with
me. The typical layout of this building, was a stairway that
led straight up to the second floor, with a door in front of
you which was the entrance to the rear apartment. If you
turned about face from that apartment, you walked down
a short hallway to another door which was the entrance to
the front apartment. All of the other doors on the hallway
were secured shut, and were part of the front apartment.
As I approached the second floor, I heard some shuffling

sounds, and then felt a sprinkling of fluid hit my face, sort of a light spray. I noticed two bare feet with a considerable amount of blood on them and blood running all over the floor. A middle aged man was standing in the hallway by the railing. He was thin, and he was naked from the waist down. He was clutching a towel to his head on the left side, which was saturated with blood, and blood was running down both arms and dripping from his elbows. He had on a white T-shirt which was also saturated with blood. All of the apartment doors were shut and there was no one else around. I approached the man and asked him to take the towel away from his head so I could see what his injury was. He had a very large gash on the left side of his head running from the corner of his eye almost to the back of his head over top of his ear. There was a large blood vessel severed which appeared to be an artery and was squirting blood straight up into the air with every heartbeat. I placed his head against the wall grabbed the towel and forced it against the large gash attempting to stop the flow of blood. I stood there holding the towel on his head trying to get the attention of the boys still on the first floor. Suddenly the door to the rear apartment opened and a raging overweight woman filled the doorway holding a broken bottle in her hand. I looked at the bottle quickly and saw that it was covered with blood. She was extremely irate and began cursing at the man. He seemed quite terrified and tried to back up further down the hallway with me still pushing his head against the wall holding the towel. It was obvious that the injury was caused by the bottle in the woman's hand and she was beginning to advance towards the pair of us indicating that he was going to get what he deserved. At that point I yelled down the stairway for the young boy to go get help from the firehouse. The woman, upon hearing this, retreated back into the apartment and slammed the door shut. She had divulged that the injured man was caught having sex with her sister when she came home. It seems she immediately went on the attack with the closest thing possible, which was a bottle on the table that she broke and stabbed the man with while he lay in bed. She tried to stab him in the face, but he averted his face from the attack and received a slicing blow down the side of his head.

In a couple minutes several fireman appeared on the stairway, asked me what the problem was, and I relayed the man's condition to them. They returned to the firehouse and placed a call for a rescue squad.

I was able to stop about 80% of the blood flow as long as I held pressure on the man's head. We stood in the hall and waited for the rescue squad to arrive. In short order, I heard the siren from the rescue out front. There was no way to treat the man in the narrow space, so I let him take the towel to walk down the stairs to the vestibule, and down the front steps to the rescue squad. I followed him down the stairs, and when he got outside I grabbed his head on both sides and pushed the towel against the wound again. We both entered the rescue squad and I continued to hold pressure on the wound as we drove to the hospital. These were the days when the paramedic service and a fire rescue squad was just a red van for transporting people to the hospital. I continued to clamp his head with a towel while we exited the rescue squad, and entered the emergency room. Upon our arrival, they took us into a room with a table similar to an operating table and had him sit down. The physician asked the nurse for some implements which she provided on a tray. He picked up a pair of forceps, because I told him that the cut vessel was an artery. When we removed the towel which was totally saturated with blood, the artery again began to squirt into the air and pump with every heart beat; he was losing a lot of blood. The doctor looked into the wound and found the source of the squirting was a severed vessel which he immediately clamped, and the blood settled down to an ooze. At that point things were under control and I was no longer needed. I had a considerable amount of blood on my skin and clothing when I went to the front desk to have them call a police car to take me back to the firehouse. We all kept several complete changes of clothes in our lockers, so we could put on fresh clothes after dirty jobs. In this case, I hand washed the blood out of everything before taking the clothes home.

I don't know what the man would have done had I not arrived on the scene. It looked to me that the woman was coming out to get him, and finish the job she had started. When she saw me tending to him and calling for help down the stairs, I think she realized the jig was up. When she started to advance out of the doorway I thought that my situation was rather precarious. I was trapped and could not retreat. To this day I am not sure how I would have handled the situation should she have decided to continue the attack. I'm just glad she didn't.

ENGINE 25

Two men in black outfits were seen walking on the roof of the building.

Engine 25 was a single engine company housed in a very early firehouse that used to have horses. Single companies usually ran two pieces of equipment. Routine equipment was usually a 1948 Ford wagon with a flathead V-8 which carried a hose and only a small booster pump, and a 1946 to 48 Autocar pumper which ran behind. The officer would ride the wagon with the driver, and the other three or four men would ride on the pumper. Of the three men on the pumper, there would be, a driver of the Autocar, a guy to work the siren and ring the bell, and the rest of the men on the back step. When they left the station the last man on the back step would have to close the door to the firehouse. The Ford wagon which exited first would usually be a half a block away by the time the Mack got started after closing the door. In the case of Engine 25 they had received a new Ford wagon in 1957, and it was a beauty. It had a front mounted pump behind the bumper, in front of the grille that was equal to the pump in the Autocar. It was built by the Hahn Fire Equipment Company, and it had an overhead valve Lincoln V-8 engine with a floor shift, and was extremely quick. It was so fast that by the time the guy closed the firehouse door and got onto the back step of the pumper, the Hahn was nowhere in sight. The Autocar driver had to know where he was going on every run because it was impossible to keep up with the wagon. The officer in the wagon would reach the fire long before the pumper, give his report, and in some cases be on the way back to the station before the Autocar pumper got there. Everyone wanted to drive it. It was well taken care of because no one in the company wanted to lose it for a mechanical repair or an accident, and get another older piece as a replacement. Drivers for the wagon were carefully selected and the piece was maintained in pristine condition. Apparatus in those days were open cab to allow full visibility, and they had no mufflers. The idea behind no mufflers was adopted because they wanted fire apparatus to make as much noise as possible to alert traffic that they were coming. The route to every fire was usually pre-prescribed so the apparatus went the same way every time, with few exceptions. One of those exceptions was when apparatus was already on a job and had finished up, and was sent to another location. When this happened there was always a danger of a collision, because one apparatus approaching from one direction could not hear an apparatus approaching from another direction due to the noise. A collision of two apparatus would usually result in multiple fatalities.

Getting back to Engine 25, I was detailed to the station for a night work, and about 3 o'clock in the morning a call came in to assist police. The address was on Front Street, a two-story business where police were on the scene as there was a report that the building was being burglarized. When we arrived, we were asked to raise a ladder to the second-floor roof, so the police could check the roof. Someone on a passing elevated train had seen two men in black outfits walking on the roof of the building, and called the police. Several police officers climbed the ladder to the roof and disappeared over the edge, and in a few minutes reappeared with two fellows dressed in black turtlenecks, black shoes, black pants, and in black face paint. Both were handcuffed, and held by the police at the front edge of the roof. When the criminals attempted to get on the ladder the police pulled them back and informed them that the ladder was for police, and not for the criminals. The criminals were led to the edge of the roof where an alley ran alongside the building and were pushed off. They scuffed back and forth against the walls of the narrow space, until they hit the ground. The police calmly climbed down the ladder, walked around to the alley, picked up the criminals, took them to the police van and put them in. It was later reported that the two burglars were roofers who had done a job a couple doors down the street. During the job they had cased this building for a burglary at a later time. They also had secreted a bar and a rope on one of the rooftops for later use. When the evening came to do the burglary, they put a ladder up on the backstreet, climbed up the ladder, and pulled the ladder up after them. They found the previously secreted bar and rope and proceeded to undo the skylight, span the opening with the bar, and lower themselves into the building. The rope was very thick and had large knots every foot for climbing. Unfortunately for them, they were seen, and their escapade was to meet an unintended end. Not only were they arrested, but they suffered injuries from their fall from the roof; such is the life of the burglar.

OVER IN A SECOND

We lifted all of the debris from the floor in large chunks and we could not find him.

This particular evening we were called to assist Engine 25, which had been sent to a fire in a furniture store. As soon as they arrived, they pulled a box alarm, and our company responded. When we arrived to the front of the building, I was told to go in the front door of the store and assist Engine 25 in advancing their lines. As I followed the hose line through the store, I came upon a firefighter who was holding the tip of the line and needed help. His name was Harry Prasch. It was very dark and we were having trouble seeing, but I knew Harry by the sound of his voice, and he knew me. I could not see any fire, but I was just backing him up, so it was his job to point the hose. We were at that location for a few minutes and we advanced a few feet, when a cracking, crashing sound was heard and a large gust of wind blew in my face. I felt the hose line shake and I yelled to Harry, "What was that?" He didn't hear me because he was gone from the front of the line. Since we were in total darkness, all I could imagine was that something had fallen and took Harry with it. Since he and I were together on the line I couldn't understand why Harry was missing and I was still standing there. I heard a lot of yelling and screaming and loud voices, everyone trying to verify if anyone was missing. When things calmed down a little, I yelled out that Harry Prasch was missing. In short order lights were stretched and the area was illuminated, and wreckage was all around. At the time I had no idea what had happened, all I knew was that I was safe and

Harry was gone. An intensive search was begun, because he seemed to be the only person unaccounted for. We lifted all the debris from the floor in large chunks and we could not find him. Eventually we got to sections of wreckage against the wall about 10 feet away. As we removed this material, there standing in a small space about a foot wide was Harry Prasch, shaking and very pale. When this section of the false ceiling had fallen, it remained connected at the top and acted like a door closing and pushing Harry with it. It stopped right before it hit the wall trapping Harry in a very small space. With all the yelling and orders being shouted no one could hear him behind the roof section pinning him to the wall. We got everything out of the way and Harry was pulled from his small prison.

It was later found that the building had been an old movie theater which was converted to a furniture store. From the outside there was no evidence it was a movie theater as the marquee had been removed. Inside, the only thing that remained was a false ceiling, and the balcony. One company had advanced the line onto the roof and pulled open a hatch and was squirting water down into the building. They did not know that that there was a false ceiling, and they were filling it up with water. At 8.6 pounds per gallon, after several hundred gallons were poured on the false ceiling it finally split and gave way. Without knowing, Harry and I had advanced to the edge of the balcony; I was still under it, and he was not. Harry was slightly forward of the edge when the ceiling came down. It broke in the center and swept down towards the walls. Harry was swept off the front of the line pushed approximately 10 to 12 feet and pinned against the wall. The ceiling was still attached at the top of the wall and was draped from its attachment point to the floor. I was left untouched because I was just under the lip of the balcony and the rest of the debris landed in the balcony and not on me. Luckily, Harry received only minor injuries, scrapes, bruises, and was scared out of his wits. It all happened in the blink of an eye, and there was no time to think or react. In seconds it was over. It's amazing how much debris 30 men can move in a few seconds. Harry was found very quickly, and the rest of us stood a roll call on the pavement in front of the building; all were present. The men from Engine 25 knew it had been an old movie theater, but when we had arrived they were all engaged in fighting the fire and there was no chance to communicate with them. Harry Prasch recently passed away, as I saw his obituary in a fire department publication.

THE WINDOW SCREEN

The screen probably weighed 100 pounds or so,
and we prepared ourselves to be struck by it.

The city of Philadelphia is full of old large factory buildings, all built around the turn-of-the-century. Since most factory work had been moved out of town long ago, these factories sit vacant and eventually catch fire, or are ignited on fire. This is the story of one of those buildings. It was four stories high, with very large narrow windows over 10 feet high. Each window was covered with an extremely heavy, mesh window screen to prevent the window from being broken by children throwing stones or any other object. Of course, when you have a fire in one of these buildings you cannot squirt water through a window screen as it will break up the stream and it won't penetrate the building. The screens must be removed from the window before the fire can be effectively fought. On this job I was assigned with another firefighter to remove the screens from the windows along one side of the building on the second floor. Part of the building was involved in fire and the order was to remove screens from the middle of the building and put some hose lines in those windows to prevent the fire from going the full length of the building. Blaise Hall and I were instructed to get 20-foot ceiling hooks off the ladder truck and pull the screens from the windows. It was definitely a two-man job because it took over 250 pounds of pull with all our weight behind it to break the screens loose from their mountings to get them down to the street. We had removed three or four of these, and had one more to go, when it happened. Both Blaise and I forced our hooks into the last screen and began to back up while pulling on the screen. In this case the screen was old and had become rotten, so Blaise's hook had gone completely through the screen instead of hooking onto it. As we pulled, eventually the screen broke loose and instead of dropping straight down to the ground as the others had done, it only dropped to the windowsill, and the top came forward towards us. We tried to hold it off with our hooks, but the area we were hooked into was so rotten that the screen began sliding down the length of the hooks. The screen probably weighed 100 pounds or so and we prepared ourselves to be struck by it. Both Blaise and I ducked as low as we could, because we wanted to take the blow across our back rather than on our heads. The screen came down full force and landed on the pair of us. I threw the screen off onto the street and after taking a blow on my back stood up and felt okay. I looked towards Blaise and saw was him attempting to pull the helmet from his head. The blow had forced it down below its normal position. He almost seemed annoyed that he had taken the blow on his head and I had taken it on my back. Since I was about three inches or better in height, he couldn't understand why I had ducked lower than he did. He felt he was injured, and since we had finished the window job we went to the officer to report that he had been struck. He was sent to the hospital for an x-ray and it was later determined he had broken his neck. It seems he took the full force of the screen directly onto his skull and his neck could not withstand the blow and broke. He recovered from this injury and returned to duty. Like most of us, he would move on to another company and work there for a while. Several years later while on vacation, he had a heart attack and died, leaving a wife and three children. He was a good friend, and was deeply missed. He was very ambitious, but like so many others I worked with he died before retirement.

THE CAT IN THE TREE

In 20 years, never once had he seen a cat skeleton in a tree.

There are certain fire companies in the city that are not very active. These are stations where older firefighters are stationed, and they remained there until retirement. The younger fellows tended to gravitate toward busier companies in more active areas. Due to vacations, sick days, and retirements, it becomes necessary to detail men from one station to another to cover holes in the roster. I was covering one such hole on a nice summer day, in a very quiet company. Usually a detail to this company was a very boring time, because the local area was filled with large single family homes and very little happened there. Sometime around one o'clock in the afternoon a call came in giving an address about four blocks from the station. When we arrived, we were met by a small crowd of about 10 people. In the crowd was an older woman in a straw hat, one or two young adults, and the rest were all children of various sizes and ages. When we exited the apparatus, the officer went forward to address the people present, the rest of us stood by awaiting orders. Since it was a local call, a ladder company and a chief were also dispatched. The officer had already recalled the ladder and chief when he went to speak to the group. He asked the group why they had called the fire department, and the old lady in the straw hat responded that there was a cat up in the branches of a tree by the curb. The older woman stated that the cat had been in the tree for two days and she was afraid that it would starve to death or die from lack of water. The lieutenant stated that he had been on the job for 20 years and never once had he seen a cat skeleton in a tree. He further stated that when the cat got hungry enough he would wend his way down the tree to get food or water, and he had no intention of removing the cat from the tree. As we were getting back on the apparatus to leave, the chief arrived on the scene. A brief discussion ensued between the chief and the lieutenant, and the lieutenant was instructed in the interest of good public relations, to put a ladder up and get the cat out of the tree. We removed the ladder from the apparatus, and placed it into the tree next to the cat. One of us put on our coat and gloves, and pulled the coat collar up and went up to retrieve the cat. After a brief struggle with the cat, which included some clawing and biting, the cat was grabbed by the nape of the neck and brought down the ladder to the ground. The fireman handed the cat to the old lady, and she immediately began soothing and petting the upset cat. We placed the ladder back into its rack, stepped up onto the apparatus, and started to pull away from the curb to a good round of cheers from the group gathered at the tree. As they cheered and waved, the apparatus backfired, the cat jumped from the lady's arms, and ran under the rear dual wheels of the truck, and was crushed. Instantly the crowds screamed at the sight of the dead cat, and began booing as we drove off down the street. Our public relations effort failed.

WELCOME HOME

They could see a large orange glow and the flickering of flames on the walls; there was definitely a fire in the house.

I was detailed to this semi-suburban firehouse for an evening shift, and as usual things were very quiet. Sometime around 10:30 PM an alarm came in giving a location about six blocks away. This was an area of large, stone, single family dwellings with large lawns and detached garages, a very affluent area. As we approached the address given, in the streetlight, we saw a man standing in the street waving us to that location. The officer stopped the apparatus alongside the man, and asked him where the fire was. The man was very excited, and he related that his neighbors were out of town on a vacation, and that he saw their house was on fire and called in the alarm. He pointed to a particular home, which sat atop a three-terraced lawn, and we approached the house from that side because there was a hydrant available at that location. The men led off with a booster line which is a smaller line on a reel located directly above a tank full of water usually 500 gallons. It took several men to advance the line up the three terraces of grass to the top level where there was a flagstone patio with comfortable outdoor furniture. Going over the patio with the hose, the men came to a glass enclosed solarium through which entry to the house could be gained. The solarium was one of those with very small panes of glass in the windows, and double doors. The line was advanced across the patio and up to the double doors where the handles were tried, and the doors would not open. Inside they could see a large orange glow and the flickering flames on the walls; there was definitely a fire in the house. The officer stood back and applied his boot to the double door handles and the doors gave way with the crashing of glass. In rushed the officer, two men on the line, and a man with an axe. They advanced across the solarium through another set of doors into the house where they stopped in a large family room with many pieces of fine furniture and oriental rugs. Once inside, they were met with a very loud scream, and an older couple jumped up from a couch still clutching their two glasses of red wine. In the large fireplace was a roaring fire reflected throughout the room by mirrors on opposing walls. It seemed the couple had returned that evening from vacation and had decided that a nice glass of wine and a warming fire would be just the thing before retiring to bed. Instantly the husband, who incidentally was a prominent attorney, insisted on knowing the reason for this intrusion. The officer in charge, stated that the company had received a report of a fire at that location, and were directed to this home by a neighbor. To prove his case he decided to produce the neighbor to offer an explanation to the irate couple. Try as he might, the neighbor could not be found, and the homeowner ordered the men with the dripping hose and dirty boots off the oriental carpets. The homeowner called police, and warned that he may be suing the fire lieutenant, so a lengthy series of reports were turned in. I'm sure the homeowner was compensated for the damage to his doors, carpets, and room. This was the same company that was involved in the cat in the tree incident, and it was another failure in public relations.

THE FIGHT

*The chief's helmet hit the floor as a result of
being pummeled about the face by a fist.*

I was in Ladder Three, when we received a call of a
house fire in the neighborhood adjacent to an elevated
train. As you can imagine elevated trains made a lot of
noise at regular intervals, consequently most people did
not want to live in close proximity to the elevated train
tracks. These dwellings were usually occupied by a low
income transient population that wanted low-cost living.
Such was the case with the property that was on fire. It was
used as a flophouse for the neighborhood toughs. Inside
there was virtually no furniture, just some mattresses that
lay on the floor upstairs, and a few chairs as you came in
the door. It appeared that no one was living in the house
permanently, as it seemed to be used for parties and occa-
sional use by a gang. We found the fire on the second floor,
where several mattresses were smoldering both in the
front bedroom and in the rear bedroom. The house had a
four- room-plus-kitchen configuration. The living room
and dining room, and a kitchen built into the shed were
downstairs. Separating the living room and dining room,
was a stairway going across the width of the house to the
second floor with a bedroom in the front and a bedroom in
the back accessed at the top of the stairs by a short step-up
landing , and another step up to enter either room. As we
were throwing the burning material out of the second floor
front and rear windows, a group of young and middle-aged
men came into the house using the front door. They wasted
no time in making their presence felt. They pushed past

people on the first floor, climbed the stairway, and stood single file near the top. They yelled for everyone present to get out of their house, and made it very plain that if we did not leave immediately they would throw us out. Our captain was acting chief that day, and he was immediately at the top of the steps where he confronted the group of men. Captain John Boos was a formidable figure standing over six feet and weighing well in excess of 200 pounds. He told the group to leave the house and wait on the pavement, and he would tell them when they were allowed to come in. Needless to say, they did not accept his order, and answered back with a few choice profanities directly at him. He again repeated his order for them to leave the house and wait on the pavement until we were through, and then they would be allowed to enter the home. I heard the conversation while I was helping throw debris out the back window of the house into the yard. I also heard the chief's helmet hit the floor as a result of him being pummeled about the face by a fist. At that point Ed Lawton who was close to the chief attacked the man in the front of the line on the steps. When I turned around, I saw the chief knocked down on the landing, and Ed Lawton and the individual who struck the chief were exchanging blows. Ed seemed to be getting the worst of it. Others on the stairway were attempting to get up into the front and back bedrooms where the rest of the firemen were to join in the fight. The firemen were encumbered with heavy running gear, big gloves, and thigh high boots which gave the young toughs an advantage, and they seemed to be very anxious to get their blows in. At the time, I was carrying a Halligan tool, which is about three to three and a half feet long, solid steel, about an inch and a quarter thick, with a large fork at one end for prying. The other end of the tool was divided into three areas: a large chisel, a flat blunt surface for striking like a hammer, and a round spike of solid steel bent down for placing into the hasp of locks to open them. I stepped up to the man who was doing damage to Ed Lawton, and clobbered him over the head with the hammer side of the Halligan tool. His mouth was open, and a large echo from the blow on his skull came out of his mouth with a loud bonk. Just after being struck his gaze turned my way and I looked into his eyes. He seemed to be staring into thin air which gave me the impression that he was already unconscious. At that instant, another blow was already on the way, and another echo came out of his mouth similar to the first one, and he started to slowly slide down onto the landing to join the captain. I remember Ed Lawton looking at me with a relieved expression on his face when his battle ended so abruptly. From the stairway, another aggressor was attempting to climb over the body of the man I just clobbered while hurling insults at me. He said something to the effect that if he got his hands on me he would kill me for what I had just done. I had the immediate reaction that I would do everything possible to keep this middle aged man from getting to me to fulfill his promise. I pushed as far as I could onto the landing sliding my feet right up against the downed men, and faced directly down the stairs at the man coming up. Again, I employed the Halligan tool when his head got into range, and clobbered him a good one. I did not hear the bonk this time as his mouth was shut, but he did get that same silly look on his face that the other man had had; however, he continued to claw his way up the stairs. I turned the Halligan around to the fork end and drew back for a first-rate defensive blow, which I struck as he seemed to be faltering. He too collapsed on the stairs, and the third individual began to admonish me verbally for striking his father on his bald head and laying him low. Throughout the short battle I said nothing in retaliation, I used all my mental energy lining up the blows, and defending the second floor from the head of the steps. The third individual found it extremely difficult to climb within range over the unconscious body of his father. He stumbled and slipped, regained his footing, and stumbled again, all the time with his eyes on me. He continued screaming and yelling at me, informing me of what he would do to me when he reached the top of the stairs. I drew my tool back again and stood at the ready, waiting for him to put any body part within range of a good solid whack, which I was more than prepared to deliver. At that point several police officers entered the house and began attacking from the first floor up the stairs, peeling the aggressors off the back of the line one at a time. That was the end of the contest, and all the aggressors were arrested for interfering with a firefighter in the line of duty, as well as assault and battery on the chief and Ed Lawton. It was later found that one of the fellows arrested was an AWOL soldier who was taken away by the military police. The two individuals I clobbered were both taken to the hospital to have repairs done to their scalps before they were arrested as my blows had cut them pretty good. I felt that the individuals that attacked us were very lucky I was carrying a Halligan tool. Had I been carrying a fire ax things would certainly have had a different outcome.

KEROSENE NOT GASOLINE

A full box alarm was pulled, because we were going to need attacks from both ends of the street.

It was after lunch on a nice sunny day, and we were out in the firehouse yard moving a couple cars around to make room for the oncoming shift. I happened to look toward the east and saw a swirling column of black smoke appear suddenly above the roofs of the buildings in the distance. I immediately knew what it was and ran into the station to sound the alarm. I told the lieutenant to look out back as he came running down the office steps. I started dressing in my running gear and so did the guys who were moving cars with me. We knew there was a fire brewing. Just then, the PA system came alive with a pulled firebox on Third Street directly in line with the column of smoke. We were on Seventh Street, only a few blocks from the fire. We headed due east as we watched the smoke column grow much larger in the distance. The fire was getting worse quickly.

The homes on Third Street were two-story, single family, brick, row homes. They all had yards in the rear divided by wooden fences, and an alleyway running the length of the block intersecting with a "T" at each end. There was access to this alleyway in the middle of the block between two homes, usually completely enclosed until you reached the start of the rear fence. It was through this entrance where we took the first hose line to attack the fire. What I saw was an inferno involving the rear yards, fences, and dormers of six homes. Since the neighborhood was in a very low income area, there were scads of trash in most of the yards which added to the fuel the fire was consuming. Dried wood fences and old shingle covered wood dormers on the back bedrooms of the homes provided enough ready combustibles to feed the fire into the inferno I saw. We attacked the fire with an inch and a half line, fighting our way out of the alleyway, but making very little headway against a really big fire. A full box alarm was pulled, because we were going to need attacks from both ends of the street, not just the middle where we were. After a few minutes, there was enough water on the fire to knock down the bulk of the flames, and we could begin to extinguish the multitude of hot spots that were still licking fire and smoking. The dormers had to be ripped to the wall studs exposing all the homes' furniture to the elements. All of the roof cornices were also removed to expose the burning ends of the roof joists. It was then we discovered the body in the yard of one home in the center of the burned area. It was in the yard near the back door of the house, somewhat in a running pose facing the door. The body was burned beyond recognition, and was identified by family members as the father of the family. They reported that he was cleaning a portable heating device called a Salamander in the yard. These devices were used at the turn of the century to heat stables and garages during the winter. Similar units are used to heat orange groves to combat frost in Florida.

This man had a bucket of gasoline, instead of kerosene, which he was using to wash out the Salamander. He was sitting on an old milk box with the Salamander between his legs sloshing gasoline all over the area and on himself as he worked. The fumes from the evaporating gasoline reached a source of ignition, and he erupted in flames, tipping over the bucket of fuel as he scrambled to get up and run. He was unable to make it into the house, and the amount of gasoline present was more than enough to extend the fire to the available fuel. What I saw over the rooftops, was the very beginning of the fire we eventually fought, with the one fatality. The metal bucket, Salamander, and center metal grid of the milk box survived the fire and gave testament to the truth of the story the family told about how the fire started.

CRASHING THROUGH THE WINDOW

*At some point the police grabbed them as the
young girl began screaming for her baby.*

It was an afternoon run, on a weekday, about 4 o'clock
near the end of the workday. We got the call, which gave
a street address, which usually meant that it was a fire. I
was the tillerman on Ladder 3 as we rounded the corner of
the street where the house was located. I had just straight-
ened out from the turn and saw no indication of any fire
or smoke on the block. Since I was in the open air facing
front I would usually be the first to see anything apparent as we approached the scene. As we slowed down to
read the house numbers I was surprised by a crashing of
glass and wood window frame on the second floor of one
of the row houses. Smashing through everything came an
older black woman in a pink housecoat diving from a room
that began to belch thick black smoke. I was aghast as I
watched her do almost a perfect swan dive to the pavement. Unbelievably, her hands folded to her sides which
made me think she was unconscious before she hit. She
landed on her head and it sounded like a coconut smack-
ing on the sidewalk as her skull cracked open and her
brains slid across the pavement to the curb leaving a wet
bloody streak on the cement. She was pulled to the curb
and covered with a yellow disposable blanket until a police
wagon arrived to transport her to the morgue. We raised a
ladder to the unbroken window and Blaise Hall went up
to break it out. The smoke that had been pouring from the
broken window changed to fire as soon as the supply of
fresh air reached the interior of the building.

Hoses led inside through the front door were driving the flames toward the windows until the water finally reached the front room. We repositioned the ladder to the window-sill, and Blaise went up and inside the front second floor room as soon as the flames were extinguished. He was inside about a minute and came gasping to the window when he found the environment untenable there. He reported that the room was filled with mounds which he crawled over going in and coming out. These were later discovered to be human remains. We were directed to the roof of the three story home to cut a hole in the roof directly over the stairway. The engine men could not make headway until the pressure was relieved from the upper floors. The heat and smoke were packing down from the top floor until a hole was cut in the roof.

We peeled back the metal covering over the roofing boards and began to attack the planks underneath. The buildings in this area of Philadelphia were very solidly built, and the roofing planks were Ponderosa Pine which was so tough that you could not drive a nail into it. We had to stitch our way along a plank by making successive cuts one behind another for eight feet, then another axe man would continue to make the next succession of cuts. After four men were spent we were able to break through the boards and ventilate the building. The last series of cuts were the toughest as smoke and fire usually poured up and out of the expanding hole.

Once the pressure was off, the hose men would proceed to extinguish all of the remaining fire in the building, and the overhaul would begin. The ladder would usually do the overhaul work as the men in the engine wet down anything that looked like a rekindle. When I got to the front room I saw what Blaise had referred to as a bundle under the window. It was a pile of burned bodies. I began to peel them apart starting with a large man on the top in a sitting position, with the rest being under his legs. He was burned beyond recognition. I rolled him up in a disposable blanket and put him into a portable stretcher. Next, I felt sick because it was a toddler burned beyond recognition except for one leg which had been well under the man's body. It still had the bottom of his pant leg, a little white shoe and a little blue sock, completely untouched by the fire. I removed his body and wrapped him up in the same fashion as the man. Under those two were two large dogs which had tried to worm their way under everything to avoid the heat. They were unceremoniously tossed out the back window into the yard. I next advanced to the kitchen where there was the body of a female which appeared to be a teenager. This body was sitting on the floor between the refrigerator and stove with her legs stretched out straight. There were large brown flesh colored bubbles on her legs below the knees, which on close inspection were imitation leather knee boots which had been heated until the gas contained in the material bubbled up to make the large blisters. She was also burned beyond recognition from the waist up. Again, her body was treated the same as the others, and passed down the stairs.

At this point the overhaul could proceed, which was shoveling the burned contents of the building to the curb for removal. I was shoveling debris out of the second floor window when a young couple rounded the corner and upon seeing the burned shell of the building began screaming and running toward the house. At some point the police grabbed them, as the young girl began screaming for her baby. I have had this sight burned into my memory for the last fifty years, and I can still hear her screaming. Unfortunately, the people burned were the grandparents, and the toddler was their son.

DON'T DO IT, DON'T TRY TO SHIFT

The groaning got louder as the apparatus
began to slip backward a little at a time.

When I was discharged from the Army I went to fire headquarters for my new assignment. I had hoped to return to my original outfit, but it was not to be. There were no vacancies in Engine 2 or Ladder 3. The individual making the assignment asked me where I would like to be stationed, while looking at a large board with engine and ladder company vacancies. I looked at the board, and did not see anything appealing, so told him he should pick. He assigned me to Engine 12 located on Main Street and Green Lane, at the bottom of a large hill near a river. In fact, the company was across the street from the river which had a sidewalk before the drop-off into the water. The company was a single engine company with a large John Bean pumper that was well used and virtually on its last legs. If you remember from before, the John Bean was a slug of an apparatus, and this was an old worn out slug. Since the company was right up against the river to the west, the local area was mostly south and east. Running east however, we were confronted with a very large climb up a very steep hill measuring about four city blocks. In order to achieve this climb the engine would have to do it in first gear and just grunt its way to the top of the hill. At each cross street there was a short landing and then the ascent would begin again until the top of the hill was reached. We were quite used to this climb as we had made it many times. We would jump off the apparatus and run ahead to the street, where we would block traffic until the apparatus passed, and then run and jump on the back step again. This is an example of how slow the apparatus was going; it was the only way to make the climb. Usually, we would be unable to make the four block climb before we were recalled by another company, and sent back to our firehouse. Responding up that hill was sort of a joke among the men stationed in Engine 12. It was also a serious endeavor for delivery trucks, let alone a fire department pumper filled with water, hose, tools, and men. It was a poor location for a firehouse, because runs to the west were impossible; runs to the east took all day, so the north and south were all that was left.

On this particular day, we were breaking in a new driver on the apparatus. This fellow thought his skills were superior, and felt he could make this old apparatus dance to his tune. We had a few calls that day which were to the south on level ground - small grass fires which we made quick work of, so the driver did very well with the apparatus. After lunch, a run came in which required the eastward climb up to the top of the hill. We started off running to the south two blocks on Main Street, and then made a left-hand turn to begin the climb. We attacked the hill on a run, and made it up to the first cross street without a problem. As usual we jumped off the back, ran ahead and blocked the street, and jumped on the apparatus as it passed the intersection. We began the climb up to the second level, and as we approached the street and leveled off, he put the clutch in and tried to shift to second. In unison we all yelled, "Don't shift! Don't shift!" but it was too late. He had already grabbed second gear, and was letting out the clutch when the apparatus stalled. We were dead on the hill. He applied the brakes, and there was a groaning from the apparatus as the brakes tried to hold the massive weight. The groaning got louder as the apparatus started to slip backward a little at a time. We had a problem. The driver quickly pulled the emergency brake, but that too could not hold the apparatus as it began its backward slide.

Down the hill we started to go, gaining speed with every foot we traveled. Everyone including the officer jumped from the apparatus, while the driver stood on the brakes to no avail. We ran behind the apparatus to block traffic on the street we had just passed. We thought there was a chance for the apparatus to stop when it hit the level area at the cross street, but that was not to be. I looked back down the hill to our last chance before calamity, the final destination: Main Street. I began a mental calculation of the width of Main Street, plus the four-inch high curb, the sidewalk, and then the plunge down the hill into the river, and wondered where the apparatus would end up. When I looked back at the apparatus I saw the driver open his door and step out onto the running board with his foot still on the brake pedal looking backward. I knew he was doing the same mental calculation we all were, and I could picture us all walking back to the firehouse with no apparatus. After the apparatus crossed that upper street it slowed somewhat, then it tilted down the grade backwards, and began to pick up speed again. We flagged down the traffic on Main Street as the apparatus continued its backward travel. By this time the brakes were groaning and squealing, and you could smell them. As it hit the level area on Main Street, the driver took his foot from the running board, and slammed both feet down on the brake pedal and pulled with both hands up on the bottom of the steering wheel, putting as much pressure on the brakes as he could when the apparatus began to slow. As he reached the curb on the far side of the street the apparatus crunched into the curb, bounced up on top of it, then stopped on top of the curb. After a short pause, it rolled forward and fell off the curb into the street. It had finally come to rest, and we wouldn't have to face the indignity of a walk back to the station. This fellow would go on to drive the apparatus again, but he never tried to shift on that hill again. One close call was enough for all of us.

THE CRASH

*Thrown out of the seat, I was unable to hit
the buzzer to signal the driver to stop.*

It was in the middle of the night when the run came in
through the PA system. It's always difficult to go from a
sound sleep to wide-awake in 10 seconds or less. This was
the case on this particular evening, at least for me, as I was
last getting to the apparatus. I got my feet in my boots,
put my helmet on my head, but only managed to get one
sleeve in my coat. It was the middle of winter, blustery and
extremely cold outside. As I climbed up onto the top of
the hook and ladder and crawled into my seat behind the
tiller wheel, I attempted to get my other arm into the coat.
As I sat in the seat, the driver, Henry Paul, was more than
ready to take off. Before joining the fire department Henry
was a professional truck driver, so it was extremely challenging to tiller for him. Where others had a problem driving large tractors, it was routine for Henry. He was very
skilled at shifting, and getting the most from each gear.
The challenging part was, after Henry had gotten the cab
around a corner, he would begin to accelerate leaving the
tiller driver in a crack-the-whip situation. The rear of the
apparatus would have to be swung out for the corner and
then quickly recovered to the straight position. This was
especially difficult if a professional driver was up front.
On this night it was to be all of our undoing.

We left the station without a problem, got to the first
corner at Seventh and Norris and made that turn easily.
The problem came at the next turn. It was a narrow street,
parking on both sides, and there was just enough room to

clear the running boards of the apparatus with 18 inches on each side to spare. Parked two cars down from the corner on the right side was a medium-sized dump truck whose rear wheels protruded out into that 18-inch space. As we approached the dump truck, I was probably eight inches or so out of line with the cab of our truck. My right rear running board behind the wheel clipped the outer dual wheel of the dump truck and rode up onto the top of the dump truck wheel. As this transpired, the weight came off my set of wheels resulting in a sudden loss of steering and me being thrown out of the seat. The rear wheels had become disconnected from the steering mechanism. The dump truck rolled forward as the running board came off the wheel. I was unable to hit the buzzer to signal the driver to stop. I have no memory of seeing anything after I was partially thrown from the seat. I felt like a ragdoll being shaken and banged into every object on the back of the truck. (What I learned recently, was that I was spun around with the steering wheel for two revolutions.) Many things were happening beyond my control, and all I could do was experience the thrashing I was receiving, oblivious to everything outside the cage I was sitting in. Eventually, after what seemed like an eternity, the apparatus came to a halt. We had traversed an entire city block before stopping. There was virtually nothing left of the rear of the apparatus where I was sitting. The entire rear of the hook and ladder truck was completely destroyed, twisted, and bent. Even the ladders had their ends bent at right angles. The only part of the truck undamaged was the plexiglass cage I was sitting in. It was a disaster. The rear of the hook and ladder was sitting on the ground; there were no rear wheels. As I climbed down from what was left of the truck, I looked back up the street, and couldn't believe what I saw. The original dump truck was slightly out of position pointed toward the curb, rear wheels still sticking out into the traffic lane. All of the automobiles parked in front of the truck were crumpled into piles of twisted metal, almost unrecognizable. Many of the houses were missing their front steps which were scattered all over the pavement in chunks. There were pieces of brick missing from the front of three houses midway down the block where the ladder had plunged into the front wall of the houses. Leaf springs from the rear suspension were lying in individual pieces bowed on the street, as was the large generator that had been bolted to the rear running board.

I don't know who told the driver that there was a problem, but Henry was totally unaware until he was close to the end of the block. He continued to accelerate and grab gears the entire way, oblivious to the damage inflicted by the rear of the hook and ladder. When everything was finally brought to a halt, and he stepped out of the cab, both he and the officer Pete Williams could not believe their eyes. What they saw was complete devastation of an entire city block on the right hand side. From the dump truck forward to the end of the block there was nothing left that was recognizable. It was almost impossible to believe that the back of the apparatus where I was sitting was capable of doing that much damage to that many objects. You saw it, but had trouble believing your eyes. In today's language you might say, it wouldn't compute. We were all dumbfounded. It was later found that we were responding to a false alarm. The officer radioed our status, being involved in an accident, and requested a supervisor. It was not very long before a host of supervisors appeared on the scene, and Lieutenant Williams was bombarded with questions and accusations. Meanwhile, a decision was made to send myself and Henry to retrieve a spare apparatus from another station where it was stored, in the northeast section of the city. A police van was called and we climbed into the back, and were driven to that firehouse to get the apparatus. When we arrived at the firehouse we found an old, old hook and ladder truck which we were to bring to the accident location. The truck was so old that the only thing separating me from the elements was a little piece of canvas flapping from the bottom of the windshield. We fired up the old Tin Lizzie and left the station on our way to the accident scene. Henry decided to take the expressway, which in subfreezing weather was very difficult for me perched out in the open with no protection from the freezing wind and biting cold. (Picture being a hood ornament on a car going 60 MPH through a blizzard.) After a frostbitten run down the expressway and across town, we finally arrived at the accident scene. By the time we got there, I needed help to get down from the ladder truck because I was virtually frozen in the seat. They let me sit in the back of a police car for 10 to 15 minutes to thaw out. It was then I noticed the pain in my left elbow, probably because my arm had been pinned to the door latch which had penetrated my elbow during the accident. Later when I got back to the station and removed my coat I found a hole in my elbow and blood on the elbow of my shirt indicating that I had suffered an injury and not realized it. I washed it off and looked at it in the mirror and there was an imprint where the latch had been embedded into my elbow, but had broken no bones, so I left it alone. Ladder 3 was restored to service in 45 minutes of transferring equipment, and we returned to the station house. That was one of the most unfortunate experiences I have ever had in my life, and after several days of pondering on it, I decided to make a move to the rescue service where I hoped there was less chance of being killed on duty. I would go on to spend the rest of my career in fire rescue till the day of my retirement. I was to find fire rescue to be one of the most fulfilling experiences in my life.

Note: The section of the city where I was stationed had very narrow streets which were designed for horse and wagon traffic. With the invention of motorized vehicles, and parking on both sides of the street, maneuvering full size fire apparatus became a feat accomplished by only the most experienced. Unfortunately, bumping or scraping a running board during a response was a frequent happening, and running at night in poor visibility made the job of tillering (steering the rear wheels, there are no brakes, just a buzzer to the cab if you need the driver to stop) much tougher. The apparatus in the accident had been reported many times for erratic tiller steering and a violent shimmy for which the apparatus had to be halted in the middle of a run to get the shimmy to stop. After reporting the same problem many, many times, the wheels dislodging from the chassis was no surprise to anyone in the company. Apparatus life in first line service was at least 20 years at that time.

MOVING

*I informed him that I would go over his
head starting with the chief.*

After the accident with the hook and ladder, and after
much thought, I decided to put in for a transfer to Engine
61. I had made the decision that since I was married, and
expecting a child, I had better seek a safer line of work
than responding to fires in the ghetto. Engine 61 was a
small single firehouse located on Rising Sun Avenue in an
area of Philadelphia called Crescentville. I transferred into
that station because I had advanced notice that they were
going to assign a brand-new rescue unit to that firehouse,
and I hoped to be able to work on that unit. It was a nice
little place with a handful of men working each shift with
just enough activity to keep us from getting too bored.
After several months, a rescue squad was assigned to that
station, and eventually I had an opportunity to work on
that unit. This is long before the paramedic program was
instituted in Philadelphia. Essentially what we had was a
red van with a stretcher and a seat inside, oxygen, some
splints, and some bandages. We were still a long way from
the intensive care cardiac units that would later come to be
stationed in firehouses.

My assignment to Engine Company 61 was not a guaran-
teed entry into the new rescue unit, Rescue 18. The captain
in that station nicknamed "Teddy Snow Crop" because of
his white hair, decided that he would use two other firemen
that he thought would be best suited for the job. I was not

selected, and became very upset that I was missing out on the experience that I had transferred into that station to get.

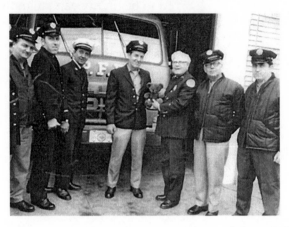

Teddy Snow Crop (presenter), Author 2nd from left

One of the guys had worked a heavy rescue before, and the other was well known by the captain as they had worked together in the station before I ever arrived there. I had an obstacle to overcome, and following my usual pattern attacked it head on. I had the advantage of knowing that both of the other men assigned to the squad did not want the assignment, and really wanted to get away from the squad as soon as they could. The captain persisted however, and they were in, and I was out, even though he knew that I had a desire to work the unit.

During the day in the summer, the captain liked to sit in the sun in a chair along the side of the firehouse and watch the traffic go by, as he got a nice tan. I took an opportunity on such a day to have a conversation with him about placing me in the squad. After stating my case, he still refused to put me in the unit, so I informed him that I would go over his head starting with the chief, and then the deputy chief; and if I had to, I would go to fire administration, and would not stop until I was placed in the rescue. He said nothing, just listened, and when I was finished I walked away leaving him in his chair to think things over for the rest of the shift. I resolved to begin my campaign the next day work, starting with the battalion chief.

When I came to work for the next day work, at roll call I found that I was assigned to the rescue unit, and that was the end of that, and my career in Fire Rescue had begun.

A BAD CHOICE

He put the shotgun against his leg...

On the first day I was assigned to the unit we got a call to a place on Rising Sun Avenue. When we pulled up to the location, I realized it was the second floor over the barber-shop that I used. There was an apartment on the second floor, and the door for the second floor was in the entryway of the storefront. There were steps going up into the front room and when we entered the apartment a grisly sight met our eyes. There was a young man sitting in a chair with his left leg extended and a shotgun on the floor. He had put the shotgun up against his leg and pulled the trigger blasting his leg into hamburger. I remember the TV set being on, and flecks of blood and meat were all over the TV screen, and every other flat surface in the apartment including the ceiling. His foot was still intact but everything from his sock level up to below the knee was missing except the larger leg bone. It looked like he had virtually amputated his own leg, which I was sure was going to happen once he reached the hospital. The police department had arrived at the location with us and the four of us stood there looking at this man moaning in the chair with his eyes closed. The fellow I was assigned with was in charge at the time. He had prior rescue experience, so he would make all the decisions. He got a sheet and wrapped the injured man's leg up with it, and to my surprise turned him over to the police to be transported to the hospital. I couldn't understand why we did not take it upon ourselves to transport this individual to the hospital, given his injury. I think the police were a little astounded that the guy in charge made that decision, but they just looked at him, and said nothing. It's in my nature to question things like this, especially if I feel the decision was wrong, but since this was my first attempt at rescue work, and he had prior experience, I let the issue pass. I immediately felt a lack of confidence in this fellow's abilities, and even with my lack of experience, I thought I could do a better job than he was doing. It seemed to me that he just wasn't interested in carrying this big fellow down the flight of stairs, and that's why he turned it over to the police department to transport. Later, I would take over that rescue squad and things would be much different. I found out from the barber on the first floor of the building, that the fellow was despondent over a draft notice he had gotten to report for duty. At that time the Vietnam War was progressing, and he indicated he did not want to go. He was afraid of getting killed. It didn't make much sense to me to amputate your leg to avoid being drafted.

DON'T GO DOWN THE BASEMENT

*He had waited until everyone had left the
home before he went to the basement.*

It was a nice afternoon in the early spring, a mild chill in
the air, and just a windbreaker jacket was needed. We were
enjoying a nice break in the weather, when the call came
in, and they directed us to a home in the Olney section of
Philadelphia. This was a neighborhood of brick two-story
row homes, which were smaller homes built just after the
turn-of-the-century to hold factory workers' families. The
police were already on location, because a family member
had called them after arriving home from a shopping trip.
She had trouble locating the grandfather who lived in the
home and usually sat in the living room. She called out
upon entering the home when she saw he was not in his
usual chair. When there was no answer, she began to look
throughout the house starting on the second floor, thinking the grandfather had turned in for a short nap. When
she did not find him on the second floor she looked out
back and out front, thinking he may have taken a short
walk. This was all outside of his daily routine as he could
only ambulate for very short distances. The light was on
in the basement so she called down the steps, but there
was no answer from the basement so she went down a few
steps and took a quick look. What she found was the same
sight that would greet me as I entered the basement. The
police on their arrival had heard our approaching siren
and decided to wait until we arrived before investigating
the basement. I was the first one down the steps where a

single bare light bulb illuminated the section of the basement toward the front. Going all the way down the steps I found it impossible to stand up. The basement was only five feet tall, and I was six feet. I looked toward the rear of the home and saw nothing, I looked toward the front, and partially illuminated in the very front of the basement, was a faint image of a person with his head bowed toward the floor. The person was behind a large pile of cardboard boxes dividing the space. As I approached, I saw there was a piece of clothesline attached to a black heater pipe which was against the ceiling. The rope was looped over the head of the old man and had constricted his neck to the point of almost severing the flesh. His body from the shoulders down was partially obscured by the boxes in the basement, so I could only see his head and neck. I wondered how a person could hang himself in a space only five feet tall. It was obvious he had expired, as his face was bright purple and drying drool was hanging from his lower lip. As I walked around the boxes to see him full on, I noticed that both hands were behind his back and had held his pant legs to keep his feet off the floor. He had gone to great lengths to hang himself in that small area, even to the point of assuring his full weight was pulling on the rope. After he had reached unconsciousness his fingers lost their grip on his pant legs and his feet fell to the floor, but his body weight still continued to pull on his neck. He had waited until everyone had left the home before he went to the basement, and set up this bizarre suicide. I don't know if he left a note, because this case was turned over to the police and the coroner to investigate. My only duty was to help hold his body up while someone cut the rope, and we lowered him to the floor. At that point we would retrace our steps and leave the house, and make ourselves available for service via radio. I never did find out why he had committed suicide, but I suspect his debilitated condition played a role in it.

As my career continued, I would see many sights such

as this, both attempted suicides, and completed suicides. Many would be much worse than this, but this would remain my first.   I was able to remain completely unaffected by it all, both mentally and emotionally. Gradually, as my work in the squad progressed, I began to feel that I was really cut out for this type of work. Most firemen prefer to do fire duty and hated working in rescue squads. The City would force them to man the squads in spite of their desire not to do it. Occasionally, someone would make the decision to gravitate toward rescue work, and eventually find a place where they could be self-sufficient and self-reliant. I began to see the value of my contribution to the service, and felt that when I responded to a call the person who needed help would be lucky that I was working that day. I made a decision to learn from every call, and advance my skills at every opportunity. If it was worth doing, it was worth doing well.

POOR ANNIE

*The smell coming from her mouth made my
eyes water and burned my nostrils.*

This is a story of Annie Hayes. I could never forget her
name, and I could never forget her story. We were all wearing short sleeved shirts on this summer day, the kind of day
when you don't mind going out on a job because you don't
have to put on coats and hats and deal with frozen weather.
Philadelphia, like many cities, is crisscrossed with train
tracks. Many streets in the city are dead-end because the
train tracks cut through them and divide a block into two
halves. This job was on such a block, a little cul-de-sac
at the end of a paved street. In this little cul-de-sac were
three frame houses, which were obviously added onto in
the years since they were built. We were motioned to enter
one of the homes that happened to be the source of the
call. I entered the home and there was a group of family
members sitting in a semicircle in the living room. Over
next to the television set was a grandmother named Annie
Hayes, and everyone pointed to her. When I asked what the
problem was, I was handed a bottle marked "ammonia",
and was told that she had drunk the bottle. She looked so
calm and serene it was hard to believe that she would do
such a thing, so I decided to check out the story. I asked
her to open her mouth wide and exhale into my face so I
could smell her breath. she did as she was told, and the
smell coming from her mouth made by eyes water and
burned my nostrils. She had indeed had ammonia in her
mouth. There was no way to determine if she had actually

swallowed the ammonia, so I grabbed a quick set of vital signs and put her into the ambulance. We took her to Albert Einstein Northern Division, where we left her in the emergency room, sure that she would be admitted. I had been looking at the obituaries over the next month, expecting to see Annie Hayes' name, but it did not appear.

The story continues almost two months later when I received a call to report to Albert Einstein Northern Division for an intensive care transfer case to another hospital in the city. Once I arrived at the emergency room, we took our stretcher, and went in to the main area of the ER and were told to wait there because they were bringing the patient to us. Down the hall came a doctor, several nurses, and two aides, pulling the stretcher. There were IV poles at both sides of the head and the foot of the stretcher, with multiple bags of IV fluid and medications hanging. Between the patient's legs was a large green oxygen bottle and tubing which led to a mask attached to the patient's face. She also had an endotracheal tube down her throat under the mask. There was a urinary bag hanging from the stretcher full of dark amber urine. After a few minutes of maneuvering we were able to transfer the patient from the hospital stretcher to the fire department stretcher, and re-hook all the paraphernalia to fire department equipment. We exited the hospital, and at the back of the squad, loaded the patient along with a doctor and two nurses and myself. The driver closed the doors, got in his seat, turned on the siren, and we pulled out of the hospital emergency room driveway, heading to Center City. Since the ride was going to take approximately 15 minutes or possibly 20, I used that time to copy the patient information from her chart. My eyes scanned the chart for the name and address of the patient, and I was astounded to read that her name was Annie Hayes, the very same Annie Hayes that I had brought into the hospital over a month ago after swallowing a bottle of ammonia. I could not believe that she had been lying in the hospital all that time suffering, with tubes coming out of every opening in her body. I couldn't imagine the amount of suffering she had gone through while I was living my life on a daily basis unknowing. Had she known in advance what was in store for her I'm sure she would've chosen another path. Again, I looked daily in the paper, and she lasted less than a week after the transfer. All the effort expended to keep her alive was totally wasted as was the transfer between hospitals. The ammonia had finished a job for which it was intended, but showed her no mercy.

BAGGED

*It looked to me that she was changing
her mind at the last minute.*

I was still working out of Engine 61, still riding the rescue squad, when one day we were called by police to an address located on a row of two-story, brick porch front homes. In front of the home was a police car with a policeman standing on the side. He had arrived there first on a call from a neighbor. The neighbor was standing with him on the payment as we arrived on the scene, and in a moment, I joined them to find out what was going on. The lady was a next door neighbor to the people who occupied the home, and they had all gone to work. She was asked to check in on the grandmother who was at home at the time alone. She was a semi-invalid due to a problem with her knee which she was soon to have corrected. She was scheduled for surgery in several days and was very anxious and depressed about it, according to the neighbor. The neighbor reported that she had gone next door, opened the door, and yelled in to the grandmother expecting an answer, and received none. She went further into the living room, called again, and again received no answer. At that point she became afraid so she retreated and made the call to the police, who called the fire department. The police officer motioned to me that we would both go inside and check out the house. The police officer mentioned in the living room that he would go to the back of the house and check the basement, and he pointed to the stairs and said that I should check out the second floor. I think he already knew in advance that whatever was to be found in the house would be found on the second floor, and he didn't want to be the one to make the discovery.

I climbed the stairs to the second floor, where all the doors to the bedrooms were closed because the family had left air-conditioning on, by way of window units in all the upstairs bedrooms, and I could hear them humming away. At the top of the stairs to the second floor was a window which overlooked the roof of the kitchen below. To the right was a doorway, so I decided to try that one first. As I open the door, a very grotesque sight greeted me; I had found the grandmother. She was lying in bed with a dry cleaner's plastic bag wrapped tightly around her head; she had suffocated. Her hands were raised and her fingernails were digging into the bag on the left and right sides as if she was trying to remove it at the last second. Her mouth was agape and the bag was sucked into her mouth; her eyes were open and stuck to the bag. It looked to me that she was changing her mind at the last minute, and was unable to get the bag away from her head or tear a hole in it to breathe. She appeared to be in the middle of a loud scream when she died, and it was horrible to look at. I called down the stairs to alert everyone that I had found the grandmother, that she had expired, and there was nothing we could do. I felt her body. She was room temperature and had obviously been that way for a time, at least since after everyone had left for work several hours before. We did not see a note lying around in the house, nor was there one in the bedroom, as is usually the case with a suicide. This leads one to think that she made the decision without a lot of forethought and deliberation. Since all suicides are medical examiner cases and therefore handled by the police and the medical examiner, we returned to the station. Later I thought that the only reason we were summoned was because the police officer did not want to go in that house by himself. He must have had a premonition of what he would discover, and set me on a path to assure that I would make the gruesome discovery.

CHANGE

Eventually, a decision was made to move the rescue squad from Engine 61 to Engine 51 located at York Road and Champlost Street. Engine 51 was located very close to Albert Einstein Northern Division Hospital, which was only a couple blocks down the street. Engine 51 also had access to several major traffic arteries leading through the neighborhood and towards Center City. It was a good decision, and gave us greater access to several new communities. When the rescue squad moved, all the men who were working the squad at the time, were asked to transfer with it. This became a sticky situation because those with seniority could refuse and compel another to take the transfer in his place. I chose to go with the squad because I enjoyed working the rescue squad, and wanted to stay in the rescue service permanently. I was happy with the move. In the end, one man on each shift went with the squad and the other opted to stay in Engine 61, which led to a 50% change in the staffing of the squad. I got a new partner whom I was very happy with; his name was John Ondik. I felt we were an excellent team. He was very good at his job, and a great partner to work with. Later, when the opportunity to go to paramedic school was offered, I accepted, and he refused. He did not want to leave Engine 51's station, and go to Center City with me. He lived locally, and working at Engine 51 was very convenient for him. He had no desire to change things, and I respected that.

PING BONK

Back and forth it went until the young
challenger missed the shot.

While at Engine 51, an interesting thing happened. I met
a fireman named Moe, who I was told was an expert at
tennis, and the pro-instructor at a local country club just
outside the city. It seemed he was also an expert at table
tennis, and occasionally someone would come into the
firehouse and challenge him to a game on our little table
tennis set up in the rear of the apparatus floor. I was told
that this would happen about two or three times a year,
when civilians would come into the firehouse to challenge
and play Moe. I had heard these were big events, where the
firemen got a big kick out of watching Moe defeat player
after player who thought he was better. Moe was in his
middle to late 50s, slightly overweight, a type of guy you
would never expect could play tennis, or table tennis, or
any sport. He just looked more like a person who would sit
in an easy chair, and read the paper with his glasses perched
down at the bottom of his nose. He looked anything but
athletic. Moe was a little sloppy about his personal appearance, and usually would have part of his shirttail hanging
out over his belt. He was a great firehouse cook and his
meals were absolutely fabulous. He was just a fun person
to be around and a great talent. On this particular day word
got around that there was going to be a match that afternoon. A player who was reputed to be a state champion
at table tennis was coming to the firehouse to play Moe,.
I happened to be there that afternoon, and everyone was
looking forward to this match. I was very excited to watch

the match as I had never seen one. At the appointed time the young man in his late 20s, early 30s, came to the firehouse with an attaché case and a suitcase. We showed him to our locker room, as he wanted to change clothes before the match. He came out of the locker room wearing a white T-shirt, white gym shorts, white sneakers, white socks, two bands of white terrycloth on his wrists, and another terrycloth band around his head. He was a perfect picture of a champion table tennis player. He opened his attache' case, and inside was a selection of what appeared to be sponsor supplied paddles. He picked one up swung it back and forth several times, swung up and down several times, and placed it back in the case. He pulled another paddle out and swung that paddle around a little bit and examined it carefully. Turning it around backward he swung it around some more and put that back in the case. Eventually after a series of trials he selected a paddle for the match, more than ready to take on Moe. While this was evolving Moe was washing dishes in the kitchen with several other fellows, since we had just finished the luncheon meal. When someone informed him that his opponent was ready, he walked out of the kitchen to the apparatus floor, walked over to the table, and picked up a paddle with some of the rubber facing peeling off and said okay. The match had begun and the ping pong ball was flying so fast you could hardly see it move. Back and forth it went until eventually the younger challenger missed the shot. Moe continued this way until the score was 11 nothing, and the game ended. The younger fellow wanted a rematch immediately, and challenged Moe to go at it again. Moe asked for a two-minute intermission, and went back to the kitchen where he selected a small, black, iron frying pan from under the stove in the drawer. He returned to the table tennis game, put his paddle aside, and confronted the young player with a black iron frying pan as his paddle. The young man was highly insulted, locked his jaw, narrowed his eyes, and seemed determined to kick Moe's ass. The second game started, and to the young man's dismay it ended the same way as the first. The only difference was 10 firemen were laughing like hell. He retired to the locker room, changed clothes, and left the station without a word. That was the last I saw of civilian tennis players coming to play Moe. I guess the word got around. I had heard these fabulous stories about Moe's table tennis prowess and would not have believed it had I not seen it with my own eyes. He must have been a very talented tennis player and instructor because the country club provided him with a house on the property to use, and his private lessons were expensive.

SPLISH SPLASH

I thought it would take a long time for her to recover from seeing what her brother had done to himself.

On this run we went to a typical block of row homes with no porches, in an Olney neighborhood. This was a case where we had been called by a young girl, who had returned home from high school, and found a ghastly sight at home. She was standing on the pavement terrified, shaking, and crying, with her hands up to her face when we pulled up. She told us her brother was in the upstairs bathroom and had committed suicide, which we found not to be the case. It was an attempted suicide. As we entered the front door of the home, arranged in a lengthy pile in the middle the living room floor and going towards the stairs, was someone's possessions. There were speakers, audio equipment, a tape recorder, boxes with things in them, and a handwritten note attached to each and every piece. What we were looking at was a bequest of a person's possessions to the people identified in the notes attached to each piece. The brother had indicated who was to get each piece, and had written a memento from him to that person, and why he gave them that individual item.

We mounted the stairs to the second floor, found the bathroom, and stepped inside, to be greeted by a mess. The brother was in a bathtub filled with water up to his chest, and colored red with his blood. The fluid was so opaque that we could not see where his self-inflicted wound was, so I reached in and pulled the plug allowing the bloody water to drain. As water drained, I found a large serrated butcher knife in the bottom of the tub, that he had used to repeatedly hack into his forearms. The left forearm had about six deep slashes going across above the wrist below the elbow. The right forearm had about 15 cuts in the same area as the left, and both were covered with what looked like calves liver, which was actually coagulated blood. He had run the tub with warm water, gotten in, hacked himself up, and swooshed his arms around in the water to prevent coagulation. He was pale as a ghost. He was either unconscious, or pretended to be unconscious, as we lifted him from the tub, and placed him on the stretcher, where we applied bandages to both arms. We carried him down the stairs, and wheeled him out to the rescue squad where we locked the stretcher in. There was no danger of him bleeding anew, or further blood loss, as he had coagulated all of his wounds before our arrival. We took him to the local emergency room where he was admitted to the hospital overnight, and discharged the next day. We were astounded that he was discharged after such considerable blood loss, but I guess it looked a lot worse than it really was considering his blood was mixed with gallons of water in the tub. I felt really sorry for his sister who was horribly traumatized by what she had found upstairs. I thought it would take a long time for her to recover from seeing what her brother had done to himself.

RAIN DROPS, SO MANY RAIN DROPS

*The only thing they could do was hold
his head above the rising water.*

It was probably the worst rainstorm we had had that year. The rain was coming down in buckets, and there was absolutely no sign that it was going to stop. I was standing at the overhead door in the firehouse looking out the window at the rain and the traffic, when an alarm came in. It was for the rescue squad only. The address was an intersection near Olney High School, so we put on our rain jackets and proceeded out into the deluge. The jackets weren't much good in the rain as they seemed to absorb more water than they shed, but we were allowed to wear them on duty. It was the only working jacket the fire department would allow you to get. As we approached the intersection we killed our siren, and began to look around for the source of the call. We left our red lights flashing so traffic could see us, if there was any. We looked up and down all the streets at the intersection, and the only thing we saw were two older women holding umbrellas standing in a puddle at one of the corners of the intersection. The sewer on that corner was stopped up, and the water had nowhere to go, and was very deep. I did not understand why the two women were together standing in the middle of a puddle towards the curb where the water was over the top of their boots. Suddenly one of them turned to us and motioned for us to come over to where they were standing. Since John was driving I elected to get out in my shoes and walk over to the women to see what they were directing me to look at. As I waded through the puddle and approached the two women, I could see a handlebar sticking up out of the water. The two women were bent over, and they were holding something with their hands, it was a human head. The head belonged to a young man who was struck at the intersection riding a motorcycle, and slid with his motorcycle into the sewer opening. The rear wheel of the motorcycle had wedged into the opening of the culvert effectively pinning its operator under the chassis so it could not be moved by either the man under it or the two women. The water had built up in that area quickly, and his yelling and screaming attracted the women who were sitting on the porch up the street watching the rain fall. They made the call, grabbed their umbrellas and raincoats, and proceeded down the street to try to help the young man who had just been struck. Finding they could not move the motorcycle, nor could they get the man out from under the motorcycle, they did the only thing they were able to do which was hold his head above the rising water. When I walked over he was almost completely submerged. Only his mouth and nose were visible and the women were struggling to keep his head up, and he was having considerable difficulty breathing without inhaling or ingesting the water from the street. Seeing his predicament I grabbed the handlebar of the motorcycle and attempted to pick it up and move it from him, which I was totally unable to do. I quickly called for the driver to help me, and he came charging through the water on a run. I quickly yelled for him to slow down, as he was making waves that sloshed over the pinned man's face and into his open mouth. Together, we were able to drag the motorcycle forward slightly, free it from the culvert, stand it up, and flop it over and away from the pinned man. I then grabbed him by his collar, which included his shirt and his coat, and dragged him away from the culvert and out into the center of the intersection where I could look him over. Once he was out of the water and was able to speak, he explained that the car had sped off after striking him, and he could not identify it due to the rain on the visor of his helmet, which was thrown from his head. He had a typical motorcycle vehicle impact injury, a severely fractured leg on the left side. He also had various other minor injuries from a slide across the intersection and being pinned under the bike. Lucky for him, in one respect, was the fact that the muffler of the motorcycle was cooled by the rainwater so it did not burn a hole into his leg, which I had seen many times before on drivers pinned by a bike. We splinted up his leg, put him on the stretcher and took him to the hospital. The two ladies went back up to the house to get a hot bath and hot toddy. They had done a wonderful job of saving the young man from drowning.

Up to that point I had never ridden a motorcycle, and after witnessing the damage he sustained from the impact I decided I would never ride a motorcycle, and to this day I haven't.

TROLLY TRACKS

To our dismay when we looked down at the young man in the street, his tibia was sticking through his pant leg.

It was a summer weekday. John and I were both sitting on the firehouse bench in front of the open apparatus floor doors. The station was located on a street called Old York Road, and there was always a reasonable amount of traffic passing by. The center of the street was cobblestones, (otherwise called Belgian blocks) and in them was set tracks for a trolley car. Up the street heading north came a grubby thin young man on a lightweight motorcycle. The light at the corner where the firehouse was located was red for him, and he began to slow down in preparation for stopping. Just like most people do on motorcycles, they hate to stop and put their foot down, so they sort of steer left and right and left and right and left and right until finally they have to stop. They're hoping the light will change and they'll be able to keep going without stopping and shifting down. He was sort of doing this back and forth wiggle type thing when his front wheel dropped into the trolley tracks and didn't come out. He tried to turn in the other direction but the wheel continued straight. He gave it a little gas and again tried to force the motorbike out of the track, while we sat there watching him maneuver. He obviously had applied a little too much pressure to the handlebars and a little too much gas, because when the wheel popped out of the track it went hard left, and he and the motorcycle went head over heels. He wound up flopped in the middle of the street between the two trolley tracks, on the cobblestones, with the motorbike on top of him. John and I got up from the bench, went out to the center of the street, and picked the motorbike up from on top of its driver. To our dismay when we looked down at the young man in the street, his tibia was sticking through his pant leg, obviously broken. We put the bike without its driver in the center of the tracks on its kickstand so people could see that there had been an accident. We were afraid if we moved it to the side they wouldn't see the individual lying in the street and would run him down. I stood by the bike waving the traffic down and John went into the station and drove the rescue squad out of the station to the edge of the street. He got out of the driver's seat and went to the back and brought a half leg splint and the stretcher over to the injured rider. We put a splint on his leg and blew it up to stabilize it, loaded him on the stretcher, and took him to Albert Einstein Northern Division Hospital. Several other firemen brought his motorbike into the firehouse for safekeeping, and we told him where he could pick it up when he was able. In this case the victim happened to be at the ideal spot for an accident, right in front of a fire rescue station. With two firemen 15 feet away, he got very quick service.

MIRROR, MIRROR ON THE WALL

Thank God there were no mirrors in that room.

It was early in the morning when we responded to a call to go to a beautiful porch front home, where the three or four occupants had not yet left to go to their jobs. Everyone in the home was quite upset. As a matter fact, one of the women was crying and had her head in her hands when we walked in the front door. It seems there had been an accident that morning. Her father, who was elderly, was going from the first floor to the second floor, tripped and fell striking the crown of his head on a step. Metal edges had been installed on the front of each and every step to the second floor, and the father had fallen striking the crown of his head on this metal. Unfortunately, he had received a horrible gash almost ear to ear across the crown of his head. Someone had applied a towel to staunch the flow of blood; however the laceration was so extensive that his face sagged, and the wound gaped open. His forehead slid down and was bunched up over his eyes, with so much skin in a pile that it almost completely covered his eyes. The covering over his skull was clearly visible. The daughter had seen it, and his disfigurement had her very upset. When I removed the towel to take a look she again looked at her father's head and screamed, and began crying all over again because of the horrible image that she had seen for a second time. Her poor father was still standing in the living room not understanding really why the daughter was so upset. Thank God there were no mirrors in that room. I'm sure that if the father could've seen the state he was in, he would probably have fainted.

I sat the man down on the stair landing, which allowed me to stand before him and work on his head, rather than him bending over. I took out some gauze from the first aid kit and dried his forehead and the top of his head, pulled off some two inch tape from the roll, and began applying it to the cut. I firmly attached the tape to his forehead and pulled his skin back up where it should have been, and taped it to the top of his bald head, reducing the size of the incision and making him look more normal. I did this in three places effectively drawing the two sides of the laceration together, and decreasing the blood flow. I then applied several compresses to the area and applied a turban type bandage to his head. We then brought in the stretcher, got him onto it, and removed him to the hospital. At least it looked a lot better to his daughter when he exited the house with somewhat of a normal face position. His cut was a quite large transverse laceration across his head, which produced a horrible disfigurement to his face, and had terrified his family members. He remained conscious during the whole ordeal, and was able to respond to commands. He also talked about his stumble and fall. Once his head was sutured shut he regained his normal appearance and went home the same day from the hospital.

BRITTLE

*I heard a sickening sound similar to
mashing a bag of potato chips.*

The city of Philadelphia is dotted with factories block after block where people manufactured many types of woven goods in the past. Most of the factories today are boarded up, vacant, and closed, because the manufacturing base has moved somewhere else. On this day we responded to a small factory building, one story in height, and inside was a group of older women going about their trade. It was obvious when we entered the building that at one time there had been many, many people working there, and now the employees were down to a handful of old ladies working in a corner. Suddenly, one of them had keeled over and her friends had called 911 for help. We arrived on the scene and it was obvious the lady had died before she hit the floor. She appeared to be in her mid eighties, extremely thin gray hair, and face powder all over her face, with lipstick. She was wearing an apron, and a pair of lace up black shoes, a nice flowered dress - the type of clothes she probably had been wearing to work her entire life. She was lying on the floor surrounded by her lady friends. We decided we would try some CPR on her, for the sake of the other ladies present, although she seemed much too far gone for our efforts to revive her. I quickly got into position to start chest compressions and the other rescue man began giving her oxygen. I placed my hands on her chest and pressed down and I heard a sickening sound similar to mashing a bag of potato chips between my hands. My first compression had broken every single rib on the left and right sides and her chest collapsed. There was nothing else to be done; she was too brittle for anything resembling compressions to work. I had to stop because her chest stayed collapsed and never rose even with the force of the oxygen going into her lungs. It was unfortunate, but she was dead beyond recovery and there was nothing that could be done for her but load her up and take her to the emergency room, where they would put her in the morgue. I looked up at the other women who were all holding handkerchiefs to their faces and eyes, and I explained that there was nothing I could do for her, and they all nodded in understanding. They all understood that she had just spent her last day at work doing what she had done since she was a young girl. It was a very sad affair, the last group of women working in the last factory in the neighborhood doing the last little bit of work that could still be produced by their old gnarled fingers.

DEAD STOP

The helmet had broken into three pieces.

The call was described as a motor vehicle accident and the address was given as an intersection. It was not far from the firehouse, probably a four-block run to get us to the location. Coming down the block we could see a large box truck stopped in the middle of the intersection and a motorcycle lying on its side near the truck. A small crowd had formed, and as usual, they were standing on the curbs on two of the corners looking on. We parked the squad as close as we could to the truck, and got out to see what was going on. The police had not arrived yet. The driver of the truck approached us first. He reported that he was driving along when the motorcycle ran into the side of the truck. A quick look around showed that the motorcycle had the stop sign, and the truck had the right-of-way, so there was no reason for the truck to stop. Obviously the man on the motorcycle did not see the stop sign, or ignored it, and continued into the intersection at the same time that the truck entered from the east. He collided with the truck, was tossed from the motorcycle which fell on its side, and wound up under the truck. He had slid to the far set of wheels, which had stopped directly on top of his head. What we discovered when we walked to the other side of the truck was his body in perfect condition with boots, dungarees, leather motorcycle jacket, and leather gloves. On his neck was a set of big black dual wheels sitting where his head should be. The first thing that came to my mind was to wonder if he was wearing a motorcycle helmet, although, the helmet would do him no good in this instance. We asked the driver to either back up the truck or move it forward so we could extract the body. By that time the police had arrived. He moved the truck about three feet and sure enough there was the motorcycle helmet with his head inside. The helmet had broken into three pieces, and it and his head, were flat as a pancake and about 1 ½ times normal size. Surprisingly, I didn't see any blood on the street as we pulled him out. Since he was already dead, the police handled the paperwork, and removed the body. There was nothing a fire rescue could do for this young man. We made ourselves available for service and returned to the station ready for the next call.

HIDDEN FROM VIEW

*I went over to the opening, lit the light,
and looked behind the paneling.*

After the move of the rescue squad from Engine 61's firehouse to Engine 51's firehouse, Rescue 18 was still responsible for pretty much the same local area. On this day we made a run to Lawndale to a home that was being remodeled by its new owner. In a neighborhood like Lawndale, when something happens neighbors are usually outside to direct the rescue squad to the place where they're needed. On this day we found the address on the street, and went up the steps to the front door of the home and knocked. A man came to the front door and told us that we would get better access going down the side of the house to the rear and entering the basement through the rear basement door. We went down about three steps, opened the basement door, and the same man was waiting at the doorway and directed us into the front of the basement where there were tools spread on the floor. The basement was empty of contents. There was a cement floor and there was paneling all the way around the basement from floor to ceiling. It was a thin plywood type paneling nailed up in 4 x 8 sheets, that appeared to have been installed many years before. Once we entered the room, we looked around and could find no one in the room, but myself, my partner John Ondik, and the man who met us at the front door. There was a stairway against the wall with a railing going up into the house, and right in the corner of the room where the stairway began there was a half a sheet of plywood missing. The man pointed at the opening and told us that there was someone in the space behind the plywood wall. The plywood wall was erected up against the front wall of the house, and there was a small space about a foot wide where someone could slide in behind the paneling. The man presented me with a flashlight and I went over to the opening, lit the light, and looked behind the paneling. About eight feet away I saw a man, who appeared to be unconscious, slumped between the wall and the paneling. I judged the distance to the man, came out of the hole, picked up a hammer, and walked down the wall to the spot where I judged the man was located. I grabbed the paneling with the claw of the hammer, and pulled it from the wall, and the man came with it onto the floor. A quick look at the man showed that he was dead. There was a large deep yellow furrow running from just above his eyebrow to the back of his head over his right eye. The yellow furrow showed no bleeding, and had an odd spiral marking impressed into it. I found out later, the mark on his head was caused by the metal covering over electrical wiring, the type seen in older homes like this one. The man was cool to the touch, deep purple in color, bordering on black. He had a small wound on his right foot and a portion of his shoe and foot were burned away. There was nothing that could be done for him. When I examined the opening he had fallen from, I noticed a large pipe going through the first floor into the basement with a large monkey wrench attached to it. It seems that the man was in the process of removing the cast iron radiators from the home, and replacing them with baseboard heat. He had attached the wrench to the black iron pipe to remove it, and obviously repositioned himself to get a good pull on the wrench. When he adjusted his position, his head came in contact with a live electric wire that had a wound metal covering over it. Ordinarily, this would not present a problem of electrocution, however, both ends of the metal covering had pulled out of their respective fastenings, and the wiring had frayed, charging the metal covering with a full jolt of household electricity.

When his head made contact, he was in a perfect position to conduct the electricity considering he had a grip on a wrench attached to a water pipe, and his foot was firmly planted on the ground. It was a freak accident, not likely to happen again anywhere. Since the home was located on a main street, I passed that house every day going home from work and always felt sad about what had happened there. Someone finished the remodeling job in the house for the family who lived there.

WOW

*There he was with a golden suntan
and a big smile on his face.*

It was a rotten winter day in January 1974, alternating between rain and sleet, and blowing hard. I had just arrived at work, had gone to my locker, changed into work clothes, and began to head for the kitchen. On the way I passed the chief's office. He was there sitting at his desk with a beautiful fresh golden suntan. I couldn't believe my eyes. I backed up two steps to the door opening, and asked the chief if he had gotten into a tanning booth during our time off. We had worked the night before and had gone home at 8 o'clock in the morning, and were due back at 6 o'clock for another night of work. I couldn't understand how the chief could acquire a suntan in that amount of time. The chief happily informed me that he had gone home in the morning and was sitting in his kitchen having his breakfast looking out the window at the sleet. He asked his wife what she wanted to do that day, and she replied she would like to have cocktails on the patio of the Bermudiana Hotel in Bermuda. The chief made a phone call and found that a plane was leaving for Bermuda within the hour and there were seats available. They quickly drove to the airport and boarded the plane arriving in Bermuda just before lunch. They took a taxi to the hotel, walked out onto the patio, took a seat in the sun, and ordered their lunch. They enjoyed their lunch, cocktails, and in an hour caught another taxi back to the airport and another flight back to Philadelphia where his car was waiting. He dropped his wife off at home and came directly to work. He changed out of his civilian clothes into his uniform and sat down at the desk to do his paperwork. The story was almost unbelievable, but there he was with a golden suntan and a big smile on his face. I believed every word, and it was all true. I knew that he had inherited a sum of money from several relatives who had died, and he could do whatever he felt like doing at any given time. I think the fire department was basically his hobby. After the story was finished, he asked me to come into the office and have a seat. He said he wanted to talk to me, and today was as good a time as any. He informed me that the Philadelphia Fire Department was starting a paramedic unit, and they were looking for volunteers. He was aware that I had a deep interest in working in the rescue squad, and he thought he would present me with the opportunity to receive more training. He informed me that the scope of the program was geared towards working in Center City Philadelphia in a mobile intensive care unit to be donated to the fire department. He said that they would form a class of approximately 20 men and send them to school to learn how to be paramedics, and administer drugs and other medications. He said the classes would be taught by staff at Philadelphia General Hospital, University of Pennsylvania, Philadelphia General Hospital School of Nursing, and the doctors on staff at both the hospital and the university. I thought it was a wonderful opportunity to acquire more knowledge, and do a better job, so I volunteered to go to the classes and to take the transfer to Center City if and when I graduated. Rescue 18 was within 20 minutes of my house, so I was sort of spoiled as far as commuting was concerned. Taking a position in Center City would require me to take a train and a subway daily to reach the firehouse where the rescue squad would be stationed. I understood that it would require a sacrifice on my part, but I was more than willing to make that sacrifice. It was one of the better decisions I would make in my life, which I never regretted for one second. Given the opportunity I would do the same thing all over again.

BACK TO SCHOOL

My partner in Rescue 18, John Ondik, received the same offer, and turned it down. That would mean the end of our working together. I did my best to try to talk him into going to school with me, but he would have none of it, and wanted to stay close to home. We lived in the same neighborhood. He was very happy at Rescue 18, and continued to work there throughout his career. I went on to attend classes at Philadelphia General Hospital with the other firefighters. I came to find out that most of the class had volunteered like myself, but several had essentially been shanghaied. It looked as though the chiefs and captains in other areas of the city had selected individuals that they were interested in seeing gone from their stations. As classes progressed, I found out that some of the students were just interested in getting out of the fire rescue service and returning to firefighting, they had no real interest in becoming good paramedics.

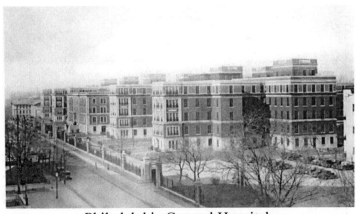

Philadelphia General Hospital

FIRST PARAMEDIC GRADUATING CLASS PHILADELPHIA GENERAL HOSPITAL

He had neglected to move the selector switch from the shock position.

Most firemen are basically happy-go-lucky, easy-going, ready-for-a-joke individuals, not serious minded students. Our most frequent instructor was a gay, male, registered nurse who had some peculiar habits. The first habit I noticed was what he did when he became annoyed with his students. He would admonish us verbally while at the same time clapping his hands and stamping his left foot on the floor. This just served to ignite a five minute round of uproarious laughter from the class. On one occasion I had the opportunity to tell him that he had a large beetle on his shoulder which caused a fit of screaming until I flicked it off onto the floor and stepped on it. This was followed by another five minutes of uproarious laughter from the assembled firemen. He was a laugh a minute. Of course, when he wasn't in the room several of us had perfected his voice, and could imitate each and every gesture that he made, to the delight of everyone present.

During one class we were being instructed by a doctor from the University of Pennsylvania on how to use a defibrillator: how to turn it on, what it could do, how to activate it, and how to recharge it after use. After the doctor had gone through several cycles with the machine, he decided to show us placement of the paddles on a person's chest. He had neglected to move the selector switch from the shock position before placing the paddles on his chest. He stood there holding the paddles on his chest explaining everything in minute detail before pushing the red buttons, one located on each paddle. We heard a loud thump, then the doctor bent over at the waist and screamed, "Jesus Christ!" It was obvious that he had just shocked himself with the paddles. They had a full charge in them, and he got hit with it all. Needless to say there was a lot of shock on the faces of the students which was quickly erased, and replaced with another bout of uproarious laughter at his misfortune. I learned from this that I should never demonstrate a defibrillator on my own chest; always ask for a volunteer.

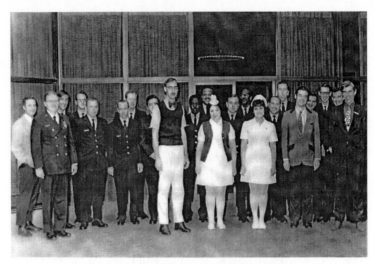

First Paramedic Graduating Classs
Philadelphia General Hospital

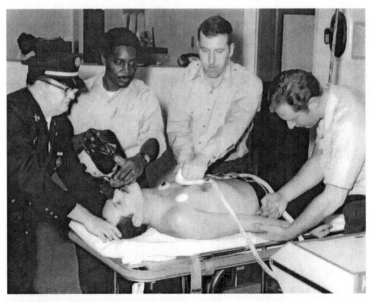

Captain Bense, Bill Pemberton, author, Ron Nyari, James
Hood (lying down)

LOOKS FAMILIAR

*I had my work cut out for me to try
to draw blood on this man.*

In order to learn how to draw blood we were sent to a ward
full of patients with no brain activity. Unlike fully awake
patients, they had no reaction to a stick from a needle, and
wouldn't move as we learned to access a vein. As chance
would have it, I was assigned to collect blood on a large,
very muscular black man, who looked like either a weight-
lifter or a professional boxer. When I looked at his arms,
they were gigantic, very thick, and I realized I had my work
cut out for me to try to draw blood on this man. I placed
the tourniquet on his arm and waited for an engorged vein
to show itself. Unfortunately, nothing appeared, and I was
reduced to probing in the bend of his arm for a vein. After
about four or five tries I was able to get blood and complete
my assignment. I drew from several others during that
morning, along with other students, and when we finished,
we took the blood to the laboratory with the vials properly
marked. As the days went on we were gradually moved
to the regular wards, and were able to draw blood from
virtually anyone in the hospital without a problem. About
a week later I was sent to draw blood on a unit I had never
been to before. I approached the first patient, a large black
man sitting up in bed reading a magazine. He was a very
large man, very muscular, and I thought I recognized him,
but of course I had never been on this ward before. He just
had a familiar look to his face as I said hello, and told him
why I was there. He extended his arm for me to prepare

to draw blood. As I looked down at the spot where I was going to put the needle, I saw several puncture marks that I immediately recognized. This was the gentleman from whom I had had difficulty drawing blood on the unit with comatose patients. I looked closely at the prior puncture marks on his arm and was able to sort out which one had given me blood on my prior attempts. I carefully inserted the needle and struck the vein right away. It was a good day for me. I couldn't help continuing to marvel at the fact that this man was sitting up reading a magazine, and had been completely comatose a week before. I was later told that the swelling in his brain had responded well to the steroids used on him.

COURIERS

Philadelphia General Hospital was somewhat of a strange place. It was dedicated to serving the health needs of many of the poor people in the city of Philadelphia. One thing I agreed with was the couriers who were hired to take messages, tissue samples, lab results, and anything else that needed to be moved through the hospital and the various departments. All of the couriers were former gang members, and other young men that had been shot in the spine and paralyzed. They were hired by the hospital to do this type work, and lived at the hospital in a ward. They all lay face down on a stretcher with large wheelchair spoke wheels at one end, which they used to propel themselves around to their various assignments. They took their jobs seriously, and they wheeled themselves up and down the hallways, and around to all the various departments which they knew intimately. They all knew each other, and they greeted each other as they passed on their assignments. They ate at the hospital, and lived there, and maintained their own society, taking advantage of the large sprawling acreage for recreation. My understanding was that they were paid for their assignments, worked regular hours, and in return, received free room and board, and any necessary assistance or medical care. The small amount of money they received in pay was more than adequate for their additional needs and wants. They were very happy there, and could come and go as they pleased during off hours. Many years later, after the hospital was torn down, I often wondered what ever happened to those fellows.

DICKEY GOES DOWN

Several immediately left the room retching.

While in class one day I made a suggestion concerning going to the morgue and watching an autopsy. The next day I was informed that we would be welcomed at the Philadelphia Medical Examiner's office to view a complete autopsy on a body. Our group reported to the medical examiner's office and was escorted to a large tiled room, with a large flat table in the center made of stainless steel. On the table was an aged female body which the medical examiner was going to autopsy, and we were going to watch. We were lined up on one side of the table and the medical examiner was on the other with a helper. I was initially struck by the fact that the room had no odor whatsoever; not what I expected. I expected either a pine scented cleaning solution odor, or a medicinal alcohol type of odor, but here there was nothing discernible regarding smell, but that was soon to change. The medical examiner picked up a scalpel from a tray of instruments and made several large incisions through the chest of the body. This was long before all the medical examiner shows on television that give you a hint of what actually goes on. Most of us had seen bodies, and handled bodies on the job, but that was scant preparation for what we were to experience here. The initial cuts were from the left shoulder to the center of the chest, the right shoulder to the center of the chest, and then down to the pubis in the center. That permitted the aide to pull all the flesh to either side and expose the internal organs. A body begins to decompose immediately after death.   We were revolted by the result of this decomposition and the presence of a sickening odor that we all found offensive. In my case, I pulled a handkerchief from my pocket and put it over my nose to block it out somewhat. Others found different methods to do the same thing, and several immediately left the room retching. The doctor looked up at us, smiled and went on with his work, which included the removal of all the internal organs, which he held up and explained. When he got to the gallbladder he opened it revealing several black and green coal like stones which he offered to the group. Of course, he had more takers than he had gallstones to hand out. This was an unexpected treat for about six of the guys standing there. This was about the time that Dickey Herbst collapsed onto the floor, and was unceremoniously dragged from the room and laid in the hallway outside the doors. He was left there with two of the other fellows who were still retching sitting on the bench in hall. Dickey Herbst would never live this down through the rest of his career, each time he met one of us he would be gloriously reminded of this event. Things progressed on through the normal autopsy until the doctor reached the head, where he made a large incision across the back of the scalp and peeled the scalp forward and hooked it under the chin. This reminded me of the poor fellow who fell on his steps lacerating his scalp whose face slid down disfiguring him. I thought at the time, hooking her scalp and hair under the chin was a great way to hold it away from the working area. A saw was employed on the skull to make a circular cut all the way around the skull, and an angular bar was hammered into the cut at the forehead level. The doctor then put his foot on a brace on the table and began pulling on the skull cap which eventually came off, and flew end over end and landed about five or six feet away on the floor. This exposed the covering over the brain, which was peeled away exposing the pinkish red wrinkled tissue. The brain was then removed from the head, placed on a separate small rolling table while an explanation about its properties and structure was given. It was explained that a fixative had to be applied to the brain so it could be sliced and examined, as this female had died from bleeding in the brain. Most of us thought that a brain sized Jell-O mold could duplicate the properties of the organ we were looking at, as it had a Jell-O like consistency. After about an hour and a half of watching and listening, we were dismissed and returned to the classroom. That was a day none of us would ever forget.

A RIGHT GUESS

*I was considered an authority on the
subject, which I was not.*

Several weeks into the class we were being instructed on the main points of recognizing heart rhythms produced by the monitor we were going to carry, and by an EKG Tracing. Our instructor, the gay male nurse, produced an image on a screen in the room, and started picking on people to identify what that particular tracing was. He picked a few people and each of them took a guess as to what they thought the tracing was, and each in turn was wrong. With each wrong answer the instructor became more and more exasperated with the class, because we had touched on this subject for several days. Finally, he asked for a volunteer to give him the correct answer to the question, and I raised my hand. By a process of elimination I thought I had deduced that the image was one of two answers which remained unsubmitted up to this point. I took an educated guess as to which one it was, and stated my answer with authority. Immediately, his demeanor changed and he seemed extremely pleased. In fact he was so pleased he held me up as a shining example to the rest of the class. He went further to say that here was a fireman who had done his homework and done it well. I thought he went too far. I had taken a guess, but I actually knew no more than anyone else who had failed to answer the question correctly, and now I was in a position where I was considered an authority on the subject, which I was not. Thank God this happened at the end of the day and we were dismissed soon after this episode, and sent on our way home. On the way out I received several pats on the back from the rest of the class, but I didn't say a word about not really knowing the right answer. I went home that evening, and decided that I would learn the rhythms or die trying. I didn't want to give up my new status in the class, and I was positive that every time someone made a mistake he would call on me to give the correct answer, and I was right. I studied those rhythms until I was blue in the face, and studied them some more. I was not going to look like an idiot in front of the class, because I knew what my classmates would have in store for me if I did. I knew that I would suffer the same fate Dickey Herbst was going to suffer for fainting at the autopsy, and I would have none of that. From that point forward each and every time I was called on to give the correct answer to an EKG tracing, I always had the right answer to the delight of the nurse. Many years later when I became a registered nurse I was still able to correctly identify virtually any rhythm presented to me for identification by other nurses, and the original training always kept me in good standing. And it all started with a guess.

LUNCH MONEY

*Evidently he had been stuffing coins in
his boots and walking on them.*

One day while we were in paramedic school, we were
assigned to work in a free clinic that the hospital ran, where
individuals could come in and receive a medical examination
with no charge for services. I was assigned a set of rooms, and
my job was to go into each room and prep the patient before
the doctor came in to see them. Usually, it was just having
them remove certain articles of clothing, or put on a hospital
gown, but this particular patient was something different. He
looked like a street person, rather unkempt, dirty, needing
both a shave and haircut, wearing an old army fatigue jacket,
a pair of dungarees, and some old army boots laced up past
his ankles. His complaint was that his feet hurt, so I was told
to get several large basins filled with a solution of water and
Betadine (an iodine solution). The instructions were to have
him put his feet in the basins to soak after removing his boots
and socks, which he did. When I went into the room carrying
one of the basins, the man had removed his shoes and socks,
and there was a horrible, horrible, odor in the room, bad
enough that I had to hold my breath as I sat the basin down.
He submerged one foot in it. As I quickly retreated from the
room, I noticed that the odor had drifted into the hallway, and
many of the staff were running for cover, all wondering what
the odor was, and where it was coming from. I quickly filled
the second basin, and walked down the hallway toward the
room taking a large breath and holding it until I had watched
him place his second foot in the solution. We probably let
him soak for about a half hour, before the doctor came to

look at the man's feet, by which time most if not all of the smell had dissipated. I walked into the room with the doctor, and stood to the side as he sat down on a rolling stool, and asked the man to lift one foot so it could be placed on a stainless steel stand used for examining feet. As soon as his foot cleared the liquid I heard a clinking sound and wondered what it could be. I soon discovered that metal was dropping from his foot into the basin. It was later found to be coins of various denominations. His leg was placed in the stand to hold it steady while the doctor looked at the sole of his foot and his toes, which were all embedded with dozens of coins that had sunk into his flesh and bone. Evidently, he had been stuffing coins in his boots and walking on them for so long they had integrated into his flesh and bone, and the reason for his foot pain was readily apparent. Once the doctor saw what had happened to his feet he realized there was nothing that could be done in the examination room. We had the man place his feet back in the basin and the doctor called the surgeon to have a look. Shortly after, a surgeon appeared and did a more thorough examination of both feet, including removal of all the coins and some rotted flesh. After his assessment, he decided to admit the patient to the hospital for amputation of both feet above the ankle as he had contracted gas gangrene and would die if his feet were not amputated. The man was placed on a stretcher, taken away to be cleaned up, and put in a hospital gown for later surgery. It was my job to get the two basins full of flesh and coins and empty them out. As I walked down the hallway past one of my colleagues, he asked me how much money was in the basins. I said that I didn't know and I was not going to count it. He then asked me if I had enough money in the basins for lunch, which at the time I thought was hilarious and so did he. No matter how gruesome a situation may be to firemen, it always presents an opportunity for a little firehouse humor. It's one of the things I loved about these guys. I left the coins in the slop sink.

DOWN HE WENT

*He started kicking back and forth trying
to free his legs from my grasp.*

Several stories come to mind when I think about my time in Philadelphia General Hospital. We had a desk in the emergency room, and we got to see a lot of things happening just after patients had come in the emergency room door. On this particular day two police officers were escorting a very oddly dressed black man. He was thin, and about six foot four. He wore some very odd clothes such as red and white wide vertical striped pants, green elevated platform shoes of about three inches, and a purple paisley shirt. He was handcuffed behind his back, and had needed some sort of medical attention after he was arrested by the police. The police took him over to a stretcher and were going to have him lie on the stretcher face up to be examined by the doctor. This fellow had other ideas, because when his handcuffs were removed he immediately struck the closest officer in the face and knocked his hat off onto the floor then promptly stepped on it. That started a melee in the emergency room between the two police officers and the patient, who initially was getting the best of both the officers since he had knocked one to the ground and was in the process of beating up on the second. I remember asking Ron Nyari, my partner, if we should get involved and help the officers, and he responded that he was not interested in getting involved in the battle. I felt an urge to get up and do something, especially since the man had his back toward me and could not see anything I was doing. I approached him cautiously from the rear as he was occupied attempting to thrash the second officer. I reached down and grabbed him by both ankles and pulled his feet out from under him. He and the officer went crashing to the floor. He started kicking back and forth attempting to free his legs from my grasp, but I had already tucked them under my armpits and was holding on very tight. They were not going to be pulled loose. By this time the first officer who had been knocked to the ground was able to regain his footing and help his partner who was in the process of getting control of the prisoner. Together, they were both able to pick the man up, and with my help, place him on the stretcher and cuff him to the stretcher. They promptly wheeled him to the back of the emergency room and secreted him in a cubicle. I have no idea what happened after that as they were all behind drawn curtains, and I returned to our desk no worse for the wear.

TOO LATE

*I saw a considerable amount of blood flow
out from under the rear door, down the rear
step of the wagon onto the ground*

The next story happened basically in the same area when Ron and I were seated at the desk waiting for something to happen. We heard sirens approaching the emergency room which we were able to identify from the sound as a police wagon. We went to the area where patients were received to render assistance, just as a police wagon was backing up to unload the patient. When it stopped, I saw a considerable amount of blood flow out from under the rear door, down the rear step of the wagon onto the ground. The two officers got out of the front, walked to the back, opened the door, and lying on a stretcher on the floor was a young black man about 17 or 18 years old with a very large gash in his neck. I saw a blood vessel showing, about as big around as my thumb which was welling up blood and spilling out onto the floor of the police wagon with each heartbeat. The boy was removed on the stretcher to the emergency room, but had pretty much lost most of the blood in his body by this time. In order to transfuse someone they first have to be typed and crossed which also requires a blood draw from a vein, a trip to the lab, analysis by the lab, selection of the blood, and delivery to the place where it is needed. All of this requires close to an hour, so the person needing the blood must be able to live on his own without it for that period of time. This young man was not going to make it that long and was subsequently pronounced dead at the scene after about 20 minutes of pumping IV fluids into his veins after clamping off the open artery. We were told that he had been up the street at an affair in Convention Hall, and had gotten into an altercation with another youth, and was stabbed. It was apparent that no one thought to place any compression on the wound to stem the flow of blood. He was probably almost bled out by the time the police arrived at the scene and moved him the one block to the ER. And the ride finished the job.

DOING GOOD

*She would agree to donate anything Life
Link could harvest from his body.*

Another story that happened in the Philadelphia General Hospital emergency room was when the police had brought in a black man in his thirties who appeared to be in a coma. The man had a heartbeat and a pulse, and a very slow respiration rate, definitely alive and warm. One of the doctors opened the man's eyes and looked at his pupils which were dilated all the way. Remarkably, the rest of his body showed no signs of injury or trauma of any kind. After giving the man a thorough examination the cause for the comatose condition was not readily apparent, and the doctors began to look further for cause. A minute inspection of his head produced a small drop of blood behind his right ear in his hair. He had received a bullet to the brain. A quick x-ray of his head showed what appeared to be a 22-caliber bullet lodged in his skull that had circled around and around inside his head until it stopped, causing the coma. By this time his family had arrived at the emergency room, and someone had been called from Life Link, which is an organ donor program that accepts donations for transplantation into individuals who are on an organ recipient list. It's a very touchy thing to approach a family whose loved one is lying in the hospital in a coma, and ask them to donate the organs to people they don't know, but that was the job of the nurse from Life Link. The nurse approached the mother of the young man in the waiting room, and began to talk to her about possibly donating his body to Life Link, so that many other people could be helped to live a more normal life free of their immediate disease problem. The mother of the patient was obviously upset, but told the nurse from Life Link that she would agree to donate anything Life Link could harvest from his body. She further remarked that this would probably be the only decent thing that he had done for anybody in his entire life. When she signed the papers Life Link took over, and removed the body to an operating room that was prepared in advance for his arrival. Very soon after, one helicopter after another arrived at Philadelphia General to remove various organs to the waiting recipients. Additionally, a series of vehicles arrived through the emergency room to carry organs to local hospitals for transplantation into another group of waiting recipients. Rumor had it that this mother's donation of her son's organs had helped 15 people in five states who received body parts to make their lives better. His mother was responsible for doing a tremendous amount of good on that day.

DO WHAT I SAY

*He came to the realization that his yelling and
screaming was having no effect on anyone.*

The next story is a lesson on how to control bad behavior
in an emergency room. The police had brought in a bellig-
erent man in his thirties cuffed, who was having a good old
time cursing, carrying on, and being noncompliant with
everything he was asked to do. He was verbally attacking
every man in the room including Ron and I who had nothing to do with him. He wanted to fight us all. He especially
wanted to thrash the two police officers who brought him
in. He hurled challenges at us all, and I sort of wanted him
to break loose to see if he could make good against two
police officers and two firemen, all four of us at least six
feet and around 200 pounds each. A seasoned nurse working in the emergency room showed us how to handle a
case like this - of a person who could not be reasoned with,
and had a mouthy tirade of curses as an answer to every
question. She asked for help in placing him on a stretcher
where she could put him in leather restraints until he came
to his senses. With our help he was placed on a stretcher
face up, and the nurse and police applied leather restraints
to both wrists, and both ankles, and placed a strap across
his chest, and fastened it under the stretcher to keep him
from sitting up and thrashing around. She then took over,
and pushed him to the back of the emergency room, placed
him in a cubicle, and drew a curtain around him. Once
the curtain was drawn everyone walked away and left him
alone in the cubicle so he could not see or hear anyone in
the vicinity. I continued to hear him cursing and carrying

on very loudly and obnoxiously for over an hour, hurling continuous abuse at anyone he thought was within earshot. Expecting to draw attention, he persisted, but it netted him not one reply from anyone. After almost an hour and a half he came to the realization that his yelling and screaming was having no effect on anyone, and he began to question if those outside the cubicle were there to hear him. His inquiry netted him no response of any kind. Even though we were listening, he had no way of knowing, because we made no noise, and all was quiet. For the next hour, he was obviously getting somewhat uncomfortable being strapped down, and he was still threatening that when he was released from his bonds, he would kick the shit out of everyone he could get his hands on. After about three hours of being strapped to the stretcher, he started developing a different tone, and was ready to make a deal. If we would let him up, and let him sit in a chair, he would let us examine him, to which he received no reply from anyone. At this point both Ron and I started to think the escapade was getting funny, because he was trying to bargain. After 3 ½ hours he was obviously in a great deal of discomfort and began to say, "Okay, okay! I get the picture. I'll be good, just let me up and undo the straps! I promise I'll be good!" to which he received no reply, and all was silent. Again, both Ron and I thought that the little nurse had him by the short and curlies, and we were quite amused at the whole thing. After about four hours of being strapped to the stretcher he was in severe discomfort and began to cry and sob and beg to be let up. His entire demeanor had completely changed, and at this stage of discomfort he was like putty in the nurse's hands, and would submit to anything to be released from his bonds. It was at this point that the nurse walked over to the curtain and drew it back so he could see that there was no one around but her. She held the key to his release, provided he could convince her that he would behave and allow her to treat his problems. The deal was struck, and the nurse informed him that any problem going forward, he would be placed back on the stretcher for another four hours, the mere mention of which started him sobbing again. This maniac was an entirely different person than the one who had originally been strapped to the stretcher and placed in the cubicle. He allowed the nurse to conduct her examination, and his further treatment was totally uneventful.

NOT OVER THE RADIO

When we got there, there were chiefs' cars parked all over the apron out front, and they were standing in the station waiting for us.

After graduating from paramedic school and receiving my certificate, I was stationed at Rescue 7 which was at 2110 Market Street. It was July 25, 1974. Upon arriving to work on the first day at the new station, I was instructed to take the rescue squad to Philadelphia General Hospital and run from the hospital emergency room where we would be working for the next six months. At the time there was no mobile intensive care rescue squad, no new equipment, no nothing, and the paramedic assigned with me and I were shocked. What we found was a broken down, dirty, piece of equipment, a far cry from what had been promised. That morning I opened the back doors of the rescue and the floor was covered with broken glass, the compartment containing the splints had several inches of water in the bottom which sloshed back and forth, and the first aid kit was virtually empty. My new partner, that I had gone through school with, Ron Nyari, was just as confused and demoralized as I was, but we took the rescue squad and reported to the driveway of Philadelphia General Hospital. We walked in the emergency room and checked in as we were instructed to do. For this we used a portable radio which one of us carried. If we received a call it would come over the portable radio. We would alert the hospital operator who would then page the physician who was riding with us to come to the emergency room where we would pick him up and go on the job. This system worked reasonably well because the doctors were young and ran very fast through the hospital to our location. I went outside to see what could be done about the condition of the rescue squad and equipment, and found that there was nothing we could do in that driveway to upgrade its condition. I got on the radio and asked the dispatcher for permission to return to the firehouse. The dispatcher asked me the reason I wanted to return to the firehouse, and I said to clean the rescue squad; it was dirty. There was silence on the radio for a short amount of time, and the dispatcher eventually came back on and said permission to return to the station was granted so we immediately left the emergency room and drove back to the firehouse. When we got there, there were chiefs' cars parked all over the station apron out front, and they were standing in the station waiting for us. It seemed everyone at fire headquarters had got into their car and drove to our firehouse to see the squad. The alarm bells were rung for the station, and every member of the company was called to the apparatus floor to get the rescue squad in shape. The night before it had rained considerably and the sides of the rescue squad up to the roof were covered with dirt from the highway. The glass inside was from an auto accident where the car windows had been broken and landed on the patient. When they moved the stretcher the glass spilled all over the floor. We got the rescue squad washed, the floor cleaned and mopped, and got the water out of the compartment that contained the wet splints. In about a half-hour we were ready to return to the emergency room and start our day over again. It was a big letdown for Ron and me to experience such a poor piece of equipment that had been abused, and run to death. Compared to the rescue squad I had just left, Rescue 18, this was a piece of crap. Rescue 18 was neat and tidy, had all equipment in perfect condition, and though it was several years old it looked new. I couldn't imagine work-ing with a piece of equipment as poor as the one we were assigned to. Later that day, when we returned to the firehouse I went up to the office, and ordered a large amount of supplies and equipment to fully stock this rescue squad. I asked the captain on duty if there was any way he could forward my requisition and get this equipment as quickly as possible. To my surprise within a day we had every single piece of equipment on the requisition delivered to us, and we restocked the unit with a full complement of good equipment. Things would change in the near future when we would receive a new mobile intensive care rescue squad that we had been promised when we volunteered for the program.

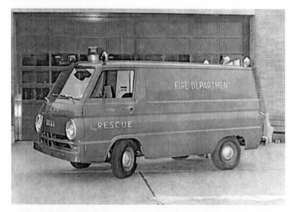

Traditional fire rescue before the new unit

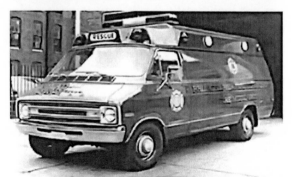

New Rescue 7 called a fire medic unit

SUNNY

He died on top of her and she could not move.

It was late evening, approaching midnight, when we were called to a luxury apartment building and directed to the tenth floor by elevator. We were given an apartment number, so we squeezed the stretcher and equipment into the elevator for the ride upstairs. When the elevator doors opened, on the wall in front of us were arrows directing us to the left, and gave us the numbers in each section of the hallway. We went to the left, down the hall, until we reached the door with the correct number and knocked. A middle-aged woman opened the door. She appeared to be extremely hastily dressed, no makeup, her hair was mussed up, and she was very upset. She quickly directed us to the bedroom where there was a large double bed with the covers all scrambled up. We found no one in the room, and turned to face the woman to ask her what was going on, when she pointed to a gap between the bed and the wall. We walked past the foot of the bed and looked into the gap which was about 18 inches wide. In that area, we found the body of a man lying on his side, wedged between the wall and the bed. In order to remove him for a better look, we had to grab the foot of the bed and slide the bed over another 18 inches, which enabled us to grab him and pull him out of the spot he was wedged into. Once we had gotten him clear of the spot we rolled him on his back to have a look. He appeared to be in is middle to late fifties, overweight with a large abdomen, absolutely dead, naked, with sperm about his penis. We asked the woman present what had happened and she gave us the following report.

The man and woman were having sex when he died on top of her, and she could not move. She reported it took her what seemed like an eternity to squirm and push her way out from under his body, which accounted for him being off the bed and wedged against the wall. In her struggle she had managed to throw him up on his side and he rolled over, and had fallen into the gap between the bed and the wall. Since there was nothing to be done for this man, we collected some information to give to the hospital as we were going to transport the body. She was able to give us the man's name and his basic information, but refused to give us her name preferring us to write down "Sunny". She did not want her name or address used in the report because the man obviously did not live there, and they were engaged in a tryst. Unfortunately, it turned into a bad experience for both of them. We picked him up, placed him on the stretcher, and removed him to the closest hospital emergency room, and that was the end of that. I did have to put down her exact address. Sorry.

GULF REFINERY

*All of the fire apparatus were consumed by
fire so there was no communication.*

Philadelphia has several major oil refineries within its
boundaries. One of the reasons for this is that several rivers
run through the city giving access to oil tankers, which
can fill up at the refineries. Even though the city is located
miles from the Atlantic Ocean, I assume the city fathers
felt it was good business to allow refineries to build on the
property next to the water. On this particular day we were
driving west on Market Street about a block away from the
firehouse, when the fire radio gave up a particular sound
announcing a box alarm, which was repeated quickly by
a second alarm being sounded and then a third. With each
alarm a list of companies to respond to that alarm follows
the sound of the alarm. Rescue 7 was announced on the
first alarm and we were at the entrance to the expressway when they called our company name on the radio to
respond. I looked in the direction of the refinery and saw
a tremendous column of smoke rising into the sky, so I
understood the rationale for pulling multiple alarms. We
accelerated down the expressway ramp and by the time we
reached the bottom we were doing at least the speed of the
oncoming traffic when we exited the ramp into the main-
stream. Upon hearing our siren the traffic started to part,
and we were able to increase our speed to a comfortable
60 miles per hour. We were instructed by radio what gate
to enter to get to the area of the refinery where we were
needed. There was a chain-link fence around the refinery, a
very large plant owned by the Gulf Oil Corporation. Inside

the fence were dozens of large metal storage tanks that contained petroleum product, each surrounded by a dike designed to handle the entire contents of that tank. Should there be a rupture in a tank, and should the product flow out of the tank, it would be completely contained in the dike surrounding each and every tank, so that the burning petroleum would not flow to adjacent tanks and start them on fire. The dikes were high enough and wide enough that each had a road built on top of it, so you could drive around every dike in the area called the tank farm.

There had been a large fire at this facility several days before and it had eventually been extinguished; however, a fire detail and fire engines were still on the premises to maintain a foam blanket over product that had been spilled

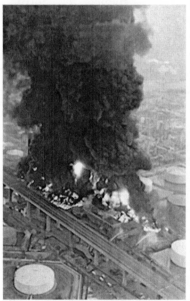

into several dikes. This was necessary until all the product had been removed from the dike and all flammable material had been cleaned up and taken away. The fire detail on location consisted of a lieutenant and a handful of firemen to maintain the foam barrier for the duration of their shift. Unknown to the lieutenant and men on location another leak in some piping had erupted, and a flammable material was flowing on top of the foam toward their location. This material was naptha, one of the ingredients in nail polish remover. It flowed silently and unseen across the top of the foam heading directly for a fire department pumper sitting on one of the dikes maintaining the foam barrier. When the flowing material reached the pumper, the ignition system on the truck caused a violent explosion, which engulfed everything between the pumper and the source of the leak. The resulting action blew the foam covering off of the petroleum product they were trying to protect, and ignited that also. The lieutenant and men instantly seeing their predicament, and with rapidly rising temperatures to over 1000° attempted to flee the area. Running along the dikes to get around the product to the exit was impossible due to the distance and the rapid rise in temperature above a level where human life was viable, left them one route to take. They plunged into the petroleum product and tried to swim through it to the other side which was the shortest distance. They attempted to stay in areas where foam still covered the material, but the fire quickly raced ahead of them and they were completely engulfed in flames and burning product. They all made it out to the road, but were burnt black in the process. All of the fire apparatus present were consumed by fire so there was no radio communication. The gulf refinery had an old Cadillac ambulance on the premises which they brought around to the administration building where the firemen lay. At that moment Rescue 7 was exiting the expressway and heading for the refinery gate which was wide open. With assistance, the men were loaded into the ambulance, and a driver who looked to be a lot older than the ambulance took off heading for the gate with the siren and lights on. As I went through the gate I saw coming towards me in the distance this old Cadillac ambulance followed by a gigantic cloud of dust, as the road was all dirt and cinders. As they drew near I could hear the roar from the old Cadillac engine, and I saw the older man who was driving. His eyes were as large as dinner plates and both of his hands were on the top of the steering wheel in a death grip. He looked terrified. When we were on the expressway we had prepared the squad to deal with severely burned people. We had all of the sterile fluid necessary to cool their bodies down effectively halting the damage sustained from superheated flesh. We emptied all of the cabinets containing these fluids, and had all the training necessary to deal with the situation quickly. How unfortunate that we never got the opportunity to assist our fellow firefighters in their time of need. We were told later that there was burning petroleum product trapped in their clothing which continued to burn them all away to the hospital. We were fully prepared to deal with that problem had we had the opportunity, but fate intervened against them. They all reached the hospital alive, but were destined to die one at a time over a period of about 10 days. The lieutenant on that job was a friend of mine that I had gone to fire school with and knew very well. In later years I have thought about this fire on many occasions, traveled the route in my mind, reviewed every minute detail, and I've come to the conclusion that I could not have done anything different, or arrived any faster than I did. I have always thought that just maybe had I gotten there a little sooner I may have saved a couple of them from their ultimate fate. I still regret not having the opportunity to have tried.

When we arrived on the location, after passing the ambulance, we pulled up and stopped under the expressway, behind a large concrete pillar. I thought I saw burning oil delivery trucks near the administration building, but they were all fire department pumpers the men had been attached to. Rescue 7 was the only piece of apparatus on the scene at that time, when all of a sudden there was a large explosion, and the top of a storage tank was launched into the air like a Frisbee. I watched it spin in the air and feared it was either going to crash down near us or on the expressway full of cars. It fell back at an angle into the burning tank it had launched from, and the air around us must have reached 500° at that point. I dove back behind the pillar for protection, and told the driver to pray that the squad did not stall out from the heat. I advised him to try and withdraw, keeping the pillar between us and the fire, which he was able to do. We set up a first aid station a good distance from the fire, and our first patient was the

Gulf Fire Chief who had a heart attack on the spot. We stabilized him, and handed him over to the next arriving squad.   It was hours before we were able to return to the fire station.   By then the whole mood of the men on duty had changed; they were remembering their fallen brothers.

CRUMPLED

*As I approached the position where the small
tree lay, I saw what we were looking for.*

It was summer short sleeve weather, and a great day to
be outside. We received a call after lunch that an individual
had been hit by a train, and we were to go on the tracks to
try to find him. The engineer on the train was sure he had
struck a person, because when he got to his next station he
got out of the car and looked at the front of the train. There
was the imprint of a body in the dirt on the front of the car,
so he knew he had struck an individual doing about 60
miles per hour. When we arrived on the scene, a gate was
opened for us to allow us access to the tracks. The tracks
were depressed below street level about 40 feet, and there
was a dirt embankment leading from the street down to
the level of the tracks. The embankment had accumulated
weeds and trees, rubbish, bottles, cans, and anything else
the public chose to toss over the fence at the top of the
embankment. The tracks themselves were clear and clean
and you could look up and down in any direction and see
there was nothing on them. As we advanced across the
tracks we looked up and down in both directions and saw
nothing visible. There were about eight sets of tracks to
get us to the other side, and then, we were confronted with
another embankment about 40 feet high. We had no idea
which track the train was using when it struck the individual, nor where he was walking when he was hit. This
was just a random search with nothing specific to guide
us, and we were not too keen on finding the body, because
these things are usually pretty gruesome. There was no

way to go up on the embankment and trudge through the four and five foot high weeds, trees, and rubbish to look for a body, so we walked at the base of the embankment looking up for any sign that something was disturbed, or disrupted. Eventually, after walking about 100 yards I noticed a small tree about the size of my thumb freshly broken. It was about halfway up the embankment, a green stick type of break, visible because the undersides of the leaves were facing towards me and they were a different shade of green than the shiny top leaves. I grasped a couple small trees and started to pull my way up the slope as it was a steep incline, and footing was uncertain. As I approached the area where the broken tree lay I saw what we were looking for. The body, after being struck by the train, was thrown about 25 feet up the embankment where it crashed through the trees and landed. He was a man past middle age lying crumpled in the brush with all four limbs at odd jutting angles. I called to my partner to stop looking, that I had found the object of the call, and instructed him to return to the rescue squad and call for an engine or ladder company to help us retrieve the body. In a few minutes we could hear the approaching company, and we directed them to the open gate so they could bring their portable stretcher over to what I had found. Since the man was dead for a long time it was a medical examiner case. Once I had pointed out where the body lay to the men on the ladder truck, we went back to the rescue squad, and made Rescue 7 available for another run. The ladder had more than enough men to accomplish the task at hand. The individual struck by the train was a street person, who appeared to be taking a shortcut across the tracks rather than walking two blocks up the street to a bridge to cross over to the other side like pedestrians should. Unfortunately, trains traveling at 60 mph are virtually silent on their approach. Their sound follows the train, it does not precede it, unless the engineer blows the horn before he approaches. Since someone crossing a high-speed rail line on foot cannot hear the train approaching, he had better be on the lookout for the light on the front of the train because that is the only way he would know that it is rapidly approaching. The role of looking both ways before you cross a street still applies when you're crossing railroad tracks. You had better be on the alert.

GOD TOLD ME

A large brown wool overcoat was floating in a
semicircle around the back part of his body

Just down the street from the firehouse on Market Street, heading west is a bridge over the Schuylkill River which runs through the heart of the city. On the east side of the river are commercial structures. On the west side of the river is a large wall that goes from below the waterline up to an expressway that runs along the water. Above the expressway is a train station. The call we received stated that someone had seen a man jump from the bridge into the river on the west side. We drove the two blocks to the bridge and I got out of the rescue squad to look over the rail into the water. There was, in fact, a man in the water up to his chest at the northwest corner of the bridge along the wall. We had to drive a circular route to get down onto the expressway and pull onto the shoulder where we came to a stop near the man's position. In a moment, a Highway Patrol car joined us, and we all got out and looked over the edge and down the wall into the water. I saw a middle-aged black man approximately 40 years old wearing a large brown wool overcoat that was floating in a semicircle around the back part of his body. His arms were out to the sides swishing back and forth as he looked up at us and said nothing. At that time a rescue squad carried 100 feet of rope, so I retrieved it from the compartment where it was stowed. I tied a knot in the end making a loop that would not slip, and threw that end down to the man, telling him to place it over his head and under his arms. The two Highway Patrol officers, my partner, and myself, began to take up the slack in the rope to pull him up onto the highway. We pulled, and pulled some more. The four of us could not raise him at all. I asked the highway officers to block the highway so I could use the rescue squad to pull on the rope and raise the man. I attached the end of the rope to the rear bumper and step so that when I drove forward it would pull him from the river. It only took a minute to make the connection and begin to pull on the rope. As it tightened we all heard a loud sucking sound. The man had been stuck in mud and sludge up to his thighs. The sound was similar to one you would experience if your boot had been pulled from your foot by mud, only louder. We did not know it at the time but the water at that location was only three feet deep, and I am sure the jumper didn't know it either. When I repositioned the squad and untied the rope, I asked the man why he had jumped into the river. He was shaking and shivering because the temperature of the water was about freezing. He had chosen the wrong time of the year to put himself in that situation. He responded immediately to my question by stating that, "God told me to jump." Of course that led me automatically to the next question presented to him, "If God told you to jump, why did you let us pull you out with the rope?" He responded, "God told me to GET OUT!" in a loud voice. I felt no need to ask another question. My partner just got in the driver's seat and headed for the nearest hospital. I found no injuries on him, but he obviously needed a psychiatric evaluation because no one in their right mind would jump into the river in the middle of the winter. When we returned to the firehouse we had a two hour cleaning job to do on the rescue squad as mud had dripped and run everywhere on the floor and stretcher. He was lucky he had picked a time early in the winter before that part of the river had frozen solid. Once the river is covered with ice, a jumper would land on it and not go through. Another platoon experienced that exact scenario two months later when a jumper received extensive fractures from landing on top of the ice.

LOOK UP

Her body gained speed as it fell the eight stories.

It was in the spring at the very beginning of our shift when the call came in. It was transmitted as an explosion about five blocks from the firehouse. An engine ladder, chief, and Rescue 7 were the first on the scene since it was in our local area. Once we arrived on the scene we were confronted with a beautiful, two-story sandstone fronted building with a prominent pillared doorway. There was a crowd of people on the pavement, and in the street in front of the building. Everyone that had exited the building was covered with a white plaster dust in their hair and all over their clothing. We received the report that they had just arrived to work and were seated at their desks when the entire ceiling came crashing down after they heard a large boom. The engine and ladder quickly went through the building and checked for anything inside that would cause an explosion, or cause the ceiling to fall in on the second floor. After a thorough search, the officers in charge decided to place a ladder against the front of the building and go up onto the roof because no cause was found inside. The first firemen onto the roof found the source of the problem immediately. There was an elderly female body on the roof, that had come out of the window of the building next door, eight stories up. As we looked up it was obvious where she had jumped from, because the window was open and the curtains were visible up on the side of the building. Her body had gained speed as it fell the eight stories, and when it hit the roof, the impact caused the ceiling on the second floor to break loose and fall on the people in the office. It's not hard to understand how the occupants felt there was an explosion given the circumstances. I'm sure everyone working on the second floor was stunned. A disposable blanket and portable stretcher were taken up the ladder to the roof, and the body was placed on the disposable blanket and wrapped up in the stretcher to remove it from the roof. The ladder company carries a wire basket in the shape of a person to be used at an event like this where a large crowd of people is assembled wanting to see everything that is going on. The body was placed in the wire stretcher already wrapped, and lowered by ropes to the ground where it was transported to the morgue. Police on the scene went up through the apartment building to investigate her apartment for the possibility of foul play, and the people covered with plaster dust got the rest of the day off from work while the offices were cleaned. Since it was unnecessary to treat anyone on the scene, we returned to the station.

ROLL BAR

A surgeon asked us to go back to the scene and see if we could recover the part which he hoped to reattach.

It was a warm summer night sometime after midnight when the call came in to respond to a depressed section of the expressway that was much below grade level. As we approached we could see the blue lights of the Police Department in the distance. It was a clear night and very pleasant to be outdoors. As usual there were large groups of police vehicles parked at weird angles, which made it difficult to spot the source of the call that had been identified as an auto accident. The police had removed everyone from their vehicles including an unconscious man lying in the roadway bleeding severely from his right hand. A quick look around told me that he had been removed from an overturned Jeep Wrangler. This small Jeep had a very large bar welded to its frame that would protect the occupants in the case of a rollover. In this case it was supporting the entire vehicle as the wheels were on the top, and the bar was on the ground. In assessing the man on the ground my partner and I noticed that a section of his hand was missing, he had only his index finger and his thumb present. The other three fingers and most of the palm of his hand had undergone a traumatic amputation. We applied a pressure dressing to his hand and an immobilization collar to his neck and scooped him up with a fracture frame, in case there was damage to his spine. We placed him on the device and laid it on the stretcher, strapped him down, and proceeded to the hospital emergency room.

When we got to the emergency room, hospital personnel

inquired if we had the missing body part in the rescue squad, which we did not. A surgeon asked us to go back to the scene and see if we could recover the part he hoped to reattach. We replaced our equipment, turned on our siren and lights and returned to the scene of the accident to search for the missing body part. Upon our arrival a tow truck was pulling the Jeep over onto its side to get it back on its wheels to be towed away. We got out our flashlights and began looking around the Jeep for the missing body part when we saw a trail of dribbled blood leading from where we found the man back to the Jeep, and a large pool of blood on the ground by the overturned crash bar on the Jeep. As a tow truck moved the Jeep, we both spied the chunk of hand on the ground where it had laid partially under the bar. The police officer present remarked that several officers had a hard time pulling the injured man from the Jeep, which may explain how his hand wound up in two pieces, since one part was trapped under the bar. The officer stated that there was a small gas leak from the Jeep and they had fears that a fire would start and he would be consumed if he remained with the wreckage. The driver of the Jeep had been thrown clear, but had not survived his injuries. We immediately responded back to the hospital with the section of hand and gave it to the surgeon in the emergency room for his evaluation. The injured man had either grabbed the bar when the rollover happened, or during the crash his hand had found its way under the bar as the Jeep rolled upside down. After viewing this accident, I made a mental note to avoid riding on the expressway in an open vehicle with no doors or roof, especially a short wheelbase vehicle like a Jeep Wrangler. I filed that with the prior note about not riding on motorcycles, ever.

POOR KID

She had jumped feet first from the third floor

Across the street from the firehouse and down the block is a short row of multiple occupancy dwellings, or in civilian terminology, apartment houses. The buildings were four stories in height, with 10 foot ceilings and had been somewhat ornate homes in the past. They had been subdivided into apartments by a past owner, and all had a large metal fire escape in the rear of the building from ground level to roof. These were mandated to allow those in apartments to the rear, a second means of escaping a fire. On this particular job we were directed to the rear of one of these buildings, with a report of an injured person lying in the yard. A quick dash through the first floor of the building put us about six to eight feet off the ground looking down into the yard, where a woman was lying amid a debris pile several feet thick. She appeared very young. She was conscious, and able to talk. I was able to climb down into the yard and reach her without much trouble to determine what we could do for her. I also had to determine how we could remove her from the yard. I immediately placed a call for additional help as her positioning created a logistical nightmare. Since there was no rear access through the building, the rescue squad had to be driven around to the side street where there was a narrow alley that ran up the rear of all the properties heading towards the yard where I was located with the patient. An examination of the young girl showed that her injuries were life threatening, and would ultimately prove to be fatal. In a suicide attempt she had jumped feet first from the third floor fire escape into the yard. She had landed on her feet, severed both thigh bones where they turn to go into the hip socket, and those bones had continued up through her body and were lodged in her intestines. I saw no other injuries other than a few scrapes and minor cuts, so we both waited for the engine and ladder to bring all the equipment for removing her from the yard. She talked to me, while we waited the couple minutes it took for the ladder to chop down the fence that separated the alley from the yard. She told me that she had no idea that committing suicide would be this painful, as she lay there shivering from shock. There was no way to splint her telescoped limbs, so we used the fracture frame to come in from the left and right sides and screw the sections together to make a device that we could remove her with. She was strapped securely to the frame, and with help we would pick her up, and hold her over our heads as we traipsed through the shit in the alley to the rescue squad. As we placed her in the back of the rescue squad, she died before the doors were closed. It was a sad day in the firehouse for everyone who made the job when we informed them that she did not make it, and died in the squad. We all felt bad that the young girl chose to die in a rubbish strewn yard with strangers. Such a waste.

TOO HOT

*Severe damage had been done. He
had a life threatening injury.*

It was in the evening probably about 10 o'clock, near
bedtime, when we responded to a highrise condo/apart-
ment unit right on Benjamin Franklin Parkway. It was one
of those buildings that people who had earned a considerable amount of money during their lifetime lived in. When
we got to the front of the building, there was a doorman
who held the door for us as we wheeled in our stretcher
with all the equipment piled on top. This was typically the
way we responded when we would not have easy access
to what we needed, and could not reach the squad in a few
minutes. We went up the elevator to the eighth floor. The
doorman had directed us which way to go when we hit
the eighth floor. We proceeded down the hallway, found
the appropriate number on the door, and knocked. The
door was immediately answered by a woman in her early
thirties who was accompanied by a young child of about
five or six, a little boy. When we entered the apartment
the very attractive young lady with long blonde hair led
us to one of the bedrooms. On the bed in the room was
an elderly man sitting back off the end of the bed with
both legs outstretched and slightly hanging over the end.
He appeared to have a pair of wet socks on, which had
slid down around his ankles in a folded pile. He also had
a wound on his left shoulder and back with a large section
of flesh missing about the size of a basketball. I asked the
woman how it happened, and she volunteered that he had
gone in the bathroom to take a shower after turning on the

hot water faucet. Without checking the temperature of the water he had stepped into the shower and began receiving a substantial scalding. Realizing he was being injured, and because of his advanced age, he became disoriented, and experienced an inability to either turn off the water, or open the door and step out. What I had initially thought were wet socks was actually the flesh on his legs from the knees down that had slid down and was piled up around his ankles. The shower was big enough that when he first experienced the burn on his back as he entered, he screamed and stepped to the back of the shower where the water only hit him from the knees down. He began yelling for help stomping up and down trying to get his legs out of the red hot water, and forgetting about exiting the shower or attempting to turn off the water. The young woman heard his cries, came into the shower, and was able to turn off the spigot, but severe damage had been done. He had a life threatening injury. In gathering information from her I had referred to the elderly man as her father, which was a mistake that she immediately corrected, stating that the man was her husband and not her father. I was embarrassed by leaping to the assumption that she was his daughter because of the age difference, so I apologized and she accepted the apology. We applied dressings to his injuries, took a quick set of vital signs and took him directly to the burn center. We had been taught that if you add the percentage of burn and the age of the patient together it would give you a rough percentage of his chance to die from the burn. The calculation is called the rule of nines which when applied to this case produced the following guess at survivability: 9% burned for each leg, 9% for the shoulder and partial back is a total 27%. Add that to his age of 80, and you have a 107% total. This rough calculation told me that he had a 107% chance of dying from his injuries. Burns of the feet are very critical, as there are many statistics from foundry workers who were burned on the feet from the spill of hot metal. It is a very serious injury, and difficult to recover from. I do not know the end result in this case. I was unable to follow it through, because it did not make the papers and the burn center was not near our firehouse.

RUB-A-DUB

The man was found on the second floor
rear, in a bathtub full of boiling water

The fire was outside of our local area, and the rescue squad that covered that section of the city was on another job, so we were sent to cover. Upon arrival on the scene we stopped near a three-story burned-out structure still steaming and smoldering from the fire that had just been extinguished. Hose lines were stretched all up and down the street and they were still charged with water. Fire apparatus were parked at the fire hydrants and there was considerable noise from the high RPMs from the pumper's motors. We had no idea why we were summoned, and assumed that one of our brother firefighters had received an injury that needed evacuation from the fire ground. When we arrived, four firemen were carrying a person towards us, so we jumped out and opened the back doors, and pulled the stretcher out onto the ground so they could place the man down. He appeared to be about 40 years old, had the features of an American Indian, with dark skin, black silky hair, and a very thick build. He was covered with wet soot and his flesh was hanging off some areas of his body denoting severe burns. He was breathing, but unconscious. With help, we picked up the stretcher, placed it back in the rescue squad, and locked it into position. I got into the back with the patient, and the driver put it into gear and headed for the burn unit. I began to examine the man, and when I shined a light into his eyes I realized he was blind because both eyes were an opaque white color. It was reported to us on the scene that the man was found on the second floor in the rear of the building, in a bathtub full of boiling water. Evidently he had sensed that the building was on fire and took refuge in the bathroom where he ran water into the tub and climbed in thinking this would protect him from the flames. Shortly, the water supply was cut off to the top floor because the fire on the first floor had melted the connections that held the copper tubing together and he lost his water supply. After the fire was extinguished, the men opened the bathroom door and found this fellow parboiled in the tub of steaming water, and called for a rescue squad. Realizing what he had experienced and what his last thoughts were before passing out, I decided to strap the man down before starting IVs. I reached in to the upper compartment and pulled out four additional straps and applied them one at the shoulders, one below the elbows, one above the knees, and one across the ankles. No sooner had I gotten the last strap applied when the man awakened, and began to violently thrash. Had I not applied the straps he could have very quickly been able to do considerable damage inside the squad. The last thing he had remembered was being trapped in a burning building and cooking in a bathtub. Being blind, he had no concept of what was going on because he could not see, and I did not know if he was also deaf. Because he was strapped down so well I had no trouble placing a large bore IV into his arm as I tried to explain to him where he was, and what was going on. There was no response from the patient as he continued to thrash. Once the IV had been started I found that his pulse rate was in excess of 120 beats per minute with adequate blood pressure, so he received a shot of morphine which calmed him down somewhat. We radioed ahead to the burn center to prepare them for what we were bringing in, so when we arrived they were ready. Initially they treated him on the stretcher, and were afraid to undo the straps until they had gotten him under control with some sedation. Eventually we were able to transfer the patient onto the hospital's equipment, and put ourselves back in service. The main reason I applied the additional straps was that I had a vision of me wrestling in the back of the squad with a large man whose skin was coming off in my hands, and I wanted to eliminate the chance of that happening.

LUCKY

*Both the doctor and nurse were covered in
sweat and at the point of collapse*

We were responding to a street that had a lot of professional offices built into row homes. As we got to the end
of the block, on the corner was a new building built where
they had torn several older ones down. This building was
three stories in height with glass doors on the front. It
belonged to a doctor, who had offices in the building.
We had all the equipment on the stretcher when we went
through the glass front door and into the lobby where
we were met by a receptionist, who directed us to take
an elevator to the second floor. As we exited the elevator we were in a large waiting room full of chairs with
people in virtually every chair waiting to be seen. Another
receptionist met us and directed us into a large examining
room where we found the doctor and a nurse doing CPR
on a large black woman. Next to the woman there was an
EKG machine that was continuing to run even though it
had exhausted the entire role of EKG paper which had run
off onto the floor in a pile. Both the doctor and the nurse
were covered in sweat and at the point of collapse from
doing chest compressions and oxygenating the woman.
The doctor looked up at us as we entered the room and was
elated to see we had a defibrillator with us, which he asked
to have charged immediately. We turn the defibrillator on
and set it for maximum, and stood by a few seconds while
it ramped up to full power. The doctor, who happened to be
a cardiologist asked for the paddles which I turned over to
him. He immediately placed the paddles on the woman's

chest and fired. While he was doing that I prepared a set of leads and placed them on the patient so we could get a tracing of what was happening since his EKG machine had long ago run dry. The monitor screen came on and we saw the flat line that comes after a defibrillation, and a good solid heartbeat which returned as a result of the shock. We immediately felt for a pulse on the patient and my partner took over ventilating the patient with our more powerful equipment. The nurse was happy to relinquish her position to a paramedic, as the doctor asked for a blood pressure. I took the blood pressure on the woman and it was almost picture book. Her pulse was also strong. The doctor was very relieved. Just then, the woman awakened and seemed shocked that there were so many people in the room. The doctor asked us to start an IV on the lady which was accomplished very quickly. He then told his nurse to go out to the waiting room and clear it of patients, canceling every appointment for the rest of the day and asking everyone to leave. As that was being accomplished, we were able to get the woman onto the stretcher still connected to the heart monitor, and with oxygen through a nasal cannula. She still wondered what everyone was doing there, and what had happened during the time she had been unconscious. The doctor tried to explain everything without telling her the whole story, about her cardiac arrest. Evidently she had come into the office complaining of a heart problem, and was in the middle of receiving an EKG when she went into cardiac arrest on the spot. The doctor had no defibrillator in the office, and had his receptionist dial 911 to which we responded, and brought him exactly what the woman needed. Had that happened anywhere else but our local area, there would have been no defibrillator available, and this woman would probably have died on the spot. She would have had to receive CPR for an extended period of time while an ambulance was called to take her to the hospital. They would be continuing with the CPR from the examining room, to inside the ambulance for the trip, an extremely taxing and difficult proposition.

When the patient was strapped to the stretcher and all of the equipment secured, the doctor, his nurse, and myself climbed into the back of the rescue squad for the trip to the hospital. The doctor bypassed the emergency room, and took us directly to a side door of one of the hospital buildings at the University of Pennsylvania Medical Center. We went through the door, where there was an elevator just inside the door, and he pushed a button to call the elevator to the main floor. The woman looked around left and right still wondering what had happened, and where she was going. I don't think she fully understood the whole picture. When the elevator arrived, we all boarded it, and the doctor pushed the button for a particular floor. When we exited the elevator we were in a cardiac unit, and the staff was waiting for him. I assisted in transferring the woman onto their equipment, and freeing up our stretcher and our equipment. We received a quick thank you from the doctor and he went to attend to the woman in an environment that he was very comfortable in. I'm sure she was well taken care of. We went out the way we had come in, reloaded everything, had the squad restocked quickly with what we needed, and made ourselves available for the next job.

OOPS

His positioning was very odd, so was the fact that his pants were down around his knees.

Round the corner from the firehouse there was a used appliance store, well known to us because it always had refrigerators, washing machines, and dryers sitting out front on the pavement for sale. We did not know at the time that there was an apartment on the second floor of the store, with access to it through a side door next to the large window in the front. We were called to this apartment one afternoon, and gained access through the door and up a long flight of stairs to the second floor, where we were directed toward the rear of this dingy space. At the far rear of this place, was a bathroom with a claw foot white porcelain tub, cruddy sink, and a toilet next to a very low window which was wide open. The window was open because it was the middle of summer and the second floor was extremely hot, as it had no air conditioning. The only windows were in the front over the store, and in the very rear, so there was not much air moving as we were in the center of the city on an east-west street. The man that directed us to the second floor told us to go over to the window because there was no one present in the apartment that we could find. He further directed us to look out the window into the backyard of the store, which contained dozens and dozens of old appliances crammed together with almost no space between them. In a few seconds I spotted the source of our call, which was a man lying on his back below the window in a small space between two refrigerators in the yard with his feet still straight up in the air, and resting against a washing machine which his heels were touching. His positioning was very odd, and so was the fact that his pants were down around his knees, and his bottom was bare. He looked like someone had pulled his pants down while he was lying on his back in the yard and his feet were elevated straight up. There was no way we could get to the man in the yard without a lot of help, so we called for an engine and ladder to assist. While we waited for them to arrive, we went back out front, and loaded our equipment in the squad. We drove around to the back of the building, and parked in a parking lot that adjoined the yard. In a few minutes we had plenty of help to gain access to our patient, who had a rather humorous story to tell. He had had a considerable amount of alcohol to drink when the urge came over him to take a crap, so he headed for the bathroom. Blind for years, he knew his way around the apartment by touch. When he went into the bathroom he turned around backwards, released his pants, and let them drop. Losing his balance slightly he staggered sideways, but was able to regain his balance without falling. Being blind he did not see that he had staggered away from the toilet and was standing directly in front of the open window. He bent at the waist and reached back to touch the seat of the toilet as he usually did to steady himself when he sat down. This time there was no seat to touch, and he had already bent too far to stand back up, so he exited the building ass first through the window and wound up on his back in the yard with his feet up in the air wondering how he got there. In about 15 to 20 minutes the engine and ladder were able to remove about 50 refrigerators to the parking lot and we gained access to the blind man for a thorough examination. As we looked him over he seemed remarkably free of injury with the exception of some back pain which one would expect after such a fall. We loaded him up on a back frame and transported him to the closest hospital for a full set of x-rays and treatment. Perhaps in the future a few bars on the window would help him remain in the apartment.

CRANDALL

When Dr. Crandall heard the orders,
he said, "That's not necessary."

The University of Pennsylvania Hospital was in our local area, and a large percentage of our patients were taken through that emergency room. One late afternoon, we received a call to go to an intersection two city blocks away from the emergency room. When we got to the scene of the accident we found the doctor in charge of the emergency room lying on the ground with his motorcycle. He was suffering from a compound fracture of the leg, and was shaking like a leaf while trying to look in control. Someone had disregarded the traffic signal and as a result Dr. Crandall was struck on the left leg by an automobile. It was a typical case for us, nothing special, so we got our stretcher out of the rescue squad put it on the street next to the doctor and quickly applied a blowup splint to his leg. Carefully we picked him up and put him on the stretcher, covered him with a blanket, loaded him into the back of the squad, and headed for his own emergency room. When we arrived in the emergency room everyone was surprised to see Dr. Crandall as the patient. We placed him on to an emergency room stretcher, and removed our splint from his leg when he was positioned correctly. A doctor walked into the room who knew Dr. Crandall and began to issue orders to the nurse in the cubicle. When Dr. Crandall heard the orders, he said "That's not necessary," after each order the doctor gave. This caused confusion, and emergency room staff all looked at one another with question marks on their faces. I'm sure they had never experienced this kind of a situation in the past. Dr.Crandall was still shaking from head to toe, and was obviously suffering from the trauma of the accident, and the damage to his leg. The emergency room personnel left his cubicle, and had a short discussion out of range of his hearing. They left him alone on the stretcher for a few minutes while their plan was hatched. After a short recess, everyone returned to Dr. Crandall's bedside for another go round on his treatment orders. This time, however, the treatment orders were given by Dr. Crandall's boss who had been summoned by the ER staff. Dr. Crandall made a halfhearted attempt to get those orders canceled, but after a stern look from his boss, he lay back on the stretcher and decided to accept his fate, which was to be treated in his own emergency room in the hospital where he was employed. One would think that he would have been overjoyed to be taken to a place where he had intimate knowledge of the quality of the care given, or maybe that's why he was terrified and shaking so much. One never knows.

PILE OF RAGS

*Walking another 10 feet on the right side of
the track was a severed human hand.*

It was late evening in the winter, and the nearest rescue
squad to us in West Philadelphia was out on a job, and
unavailable. In this eventuality, it was our responsibility
to respond to any jobs they were unable to take. On this
evening, we received an address south of an intersection of
two streets, a good distance from our firehouse. When we
arrived on location, the street was darkened, and we were
sitting under a railroad bridge looking for the source of
the call. I asked fire radio for a better address at this location, and immediately, they responded asking me if I saw
a railroad bridge. I reported that I was parked underneath
the bridge, and was instructed that the call came from a
passenger locomotive engineer who was sure he had struck
a person walking across the bridge that evening. I asked
my partner to wait in the squad while I investigated the call
by climbing up an embankment so I could see the railroad
tracks. As with most railroad embankments it was littered
with tin cans, trash, papers, and all manner of debris,
which I stumbled over with each step. After much struggle
I reached the top of the embankment and had a view up and
down the railroad tracks. I was well aware that a speeding
train made no noise in advance of its arrival to my location, and was on the lookout up and down the track for the
light on the front of any approaching train. Seeing the light
would give me the only warning to get off the track before
the trains arrival at 60 miles per hour. As I walked across
the bridge, I shined my light from left to right, and about

30 feet into the search I spotted a pair of tied sneakers sitting together on the trestle. Naturally I wondered why someone would place their sneakers together on the train trestle and why the laces were still tied. I had a tough time putting the entire picture together and arriving at a sensible conclusion. I moved on across the trestle heading toward the embankment on the other side of the street where the rescue was parked. Another 10 feet down the right side of the track I spotted a severed human hand that the train had run over. It still remained on the track with the fingers draped over the outside. I knew I would find something ugly a little further on. About another 30 feet away was a large circular bundle of clothing that resembled a torn and punctured wool winter coat and some other fabrics all ripped, torn, and pierced. I shined a light close and bent over to examine it thoroughly. It was about knee-high and I saw no signs of body parts or a person until I moved it with my foot. There was the body all rolled up in a ball inside the coat. I could not tell age or sex; all I could see were bloody bones and torn clothing. I left that bundle, and walked across the rest of the track and spotted nothing, all the while keeping an eye out for an approaching train, as I did not want to get caught on the trestle like the person I found. I contacted fire radio and related to them what I had found on the track, and informed them that there was no need for fire rescue at this point. I was ordered to stay in position. Alternative transportation was en route to pick up the body, and I was to show them what I had found. This would not be the first time that I would find tied footwear sitting together after the occupant had had them blown from their feet. I would see an alley full of fire Department boots sitting the same way after the men had been blown from them in an explosion.

YELLOW CADILLAC

As we drove down the expressway there
was no sign that anything was wrong.

It was a nice summer evening, one of those evenings
where you could drive around with your windows down
on the expressway just enjoying the warm weather. We
received a call to respond to an accident on the expressway. These were usually large affairs with many police
cars around multicar accidents. There would be lots of
flashing lights and people to direct you to the spot you
were needed. In this case we went above the location and
entered the expressway because the accident was supposed
to be in the southbound lanes. As we drove down the
expressway there was no sign that anything was wrong
and only one vehicle sitting on the shoulder of the road,
so we pulled up behind it and parked. Leaving our emergency lights on, I got out of the vehicle and approached
the man sitting in the driver's seat of the car, which was a
brand spanking new Cadillac Coupe Deville in a beautiful yellow color. The car was completely destroyed: the
roof was caved in, the windows were broken, the hood and
trunk were smashed and wrinkled, so were the doors, and
both mirrors were off. It was just an absolute mess. Sitting
in the driver's seat was an older black man who had an
injury to his lower lip where one of his teeth had punctured through and was visible. As I questioned the man
about any injuries, I could smell whiskey spilled all over
the inside of the car, and the man appeared intoxicated.
Since the car was completely destroyed, I looked around
for the other vehicles involved in the collision, but this was

the only car on the road. I couldn't understand how the car had become so damaged without any other cars, trucks, or anything else involved in the accident, just this one car. The accident appeared fresh because there was steam still coming from the hood of the car, and the dash lights inside were still lit. Everything appeared as though the accident had just happened. The part of the expressway we were sitting on runs alongside the Schuylkill River on the west side, and on the east side is a very high angled stone façade that had been carved away enough to make the road. Over the expressway were bridges which had to be accessed by leaving the expressway and going up a ramp to the cross street where you would be forced to turn left or right after stopping. The driver of this car, being drunk, exited the expressway, headed up the ramp, did not stop, plowed through the retaining rail, and launched the car into midair. When the car came to rest it landed on its wheels, but the angle of the cliff would not sustain its position, and it began to roll. The car rolled side over side many times down the cliff until it came to rest on the shoulder of the expressway wheels down with the driver still inside. It was a single car accident with two remarkable occurrences. One, the man was only slightly injured from the frontal impact; two, the vehicle landed square on its wheels giving the impression that it had been pulled over and parked on the shoulder of the expressway. We removed the man from the driver's seat, placed him on our stretcher, and loaded him into the rescue squad. We took him to the hospital to be treated for the only injury we saw, which was the hole in his lip that had been punctured by a jagged lower tooth.

DOCTOR?

*Some of his orders gave incorrect doses,
and others incorrect medications*

It was another run to one of the luxury apartment houses bordering the Benjamin Franklin Parkway. Once we arrived under the portico at the front of the building, a doorman was waiting. He held the door open, directed us to a particular elevator, and gave us an apartment number. As we walked down the hallway with the equipment at a quick pace, someone came out of the apartment and directed us inside, where we found an older woman on the floor, obviously in cardiac arrest. As usual, we began our chest compressions, and oxygenating the woman, when a younger man at the location identified himself as a physician, and wanted to assume responsibility for managing this case. He informed us that he was the son of the woman, and he asked us if we carried particular medications in our drug box and we told him we did. One thing that struck us as odd was that no one was performing CPR on the patient before our arrival, especially with a doctor present on the scene. We were able to get an IV started quickly and he began to tell us what medications he wanted us to administer; however, some of his orders gave incorrect doses, and others incorrect medications. We were functioning under a protocol which allowed us to use certain medications, certain doses, and in a specified order of administration. I informed the doctor that this was the case, but he insisted that we administer what he was ordering, which made me suspicious. A brief conversation ensued about his orders, and a decision was made to follow our protocol, and as quickly as possible remove the woman from the apartment to the hospital. Things were not going well, and we were in conflict with the son of the patient, and the problem was escalating quickly. We did everything we could for the patient en route to the hospital, but her condition was showing no signs of improvement. We had called ahead stating we had a cardiac arrest on board, and they were ready for us when we arrived at the hospital. When we removed the patient from our stretcher in the procedure room, I overheard the son of the patient explain to the emergency room physician that he was a doctor. The emergency room physician asked him what his specialty was, and he replied that he was a podiatrist. His answer explained a lot, especially the fact that he was virtually clueless with regard to cardiac medications, doses, and application; and probably should not have interfered in our treatment of his mother who did not recover from her condition. This was the second time that our care had been interfered with by a physician who had virtually no idea of how to treat a cardiac condition. Both of the individuals had ordered wrong medications, wrong doses, and lied about their experience, or withheld information from us about their credentials. From these experiences, a realization surfaced in my mind that 50% of all physicians graduated in the bottom half of their class, so I became very wary of strangers wanting to practice medicine on people who were not their patients and had not given them consent. We had trouble processing the realization that he was committing malpractice on his own mother.

DRAIN CLEANER

He presented somewhat like a circus contortionist,
with his limbs folded in different directions.

This is a story about an accident at Children's Hospital
in Philadelphia - about a repairman who was severely
injured while working on a drain at the underground parking garage. On this particular day just after a rain, one of
the drainage grates in the garage had a problem keeping
the water away from a ramp. This drain was at the top of
the ramp used to exit the underground garage. Before he
began work on the drain in the center of the driveway at
the top of the ramp, he placed barricades across that particular exit so no one would use that ramp, and put him in
danger. The garage had several ramps by which cars could
exit, so this was an inconvenience to no one. The workman
had removed the grating from the drain and was cleaning
out material which had collected, to allow proper drainage.
Down below the ramp, underground, someone had decided
she had to use that particular exit so she got out of her car
and moved the barricade to the side so she could enter the
upward ramp. As she drove up the ramp to the very top she
could not see the workman on his hands and knees in front
of the drain. She drove the car up the ramp rather quickly,
and drove over top of the kneeling workman crushing
him under the car. The driver continued to drive on, and
other people on the scene stopped her as she was exiting
onto the street. We were called to the scene, and found the
workman lying at the top of the ramp in shock, one of his
legs was broken at the hip and turned in such a fashion
that his ankle rested alongside his ear. When I looked at

him, I saw he was holding his ankle with one hand and the other hand rested in a weird position because the arm was broken. The left leg was also broken and folded up under his buttocks in a very unnatural position. He presented somewhat like a circus contortionist with his limbs folded in different directions. I made a decision not to attempt to move anything, since he had no open fractures, and I did not see a lot of swelling indicating blood loss into the tissues. We brought out our fracture frame that breaks in half, forming a scoop coming in from each side and reattaching at each end. We used this device to pick him up in exactly the position that he was in on the ground without moving or twisting anything. We picked the fracture frame up, placed it on our stretcher, and removed him to the University of Pennsylvania Hospital emergency room. Since we radioed ahead to the emergency room the condition of our patient, they had an orthopedic doctor waiting to assess him when we arrived. We were able to place him on a table in the emergency room and disconnect our fracture frame leaving him in the exact position he was in at the accident scene. The orthopedic surgeon walked around the table very carefully looking at every angle his limbs were twisted in, and after a few minutes of taking mental notes he decided his course of action. I was thinking along the lines of him ordering x-rays before he attempted to move any of the joints, but I was surprised when he grabbed a leg and began to manipulate it back into its original position. He proceeded very quickly taking only a few seconds to move each limb back where they belonged, and giving the man a totally reconstructed look like he had never ever been injured in the first place. I was absolutely amazed to see how well he looked lying there without so much as a finger out of place. He looked like he could get up off the stretcher and walk away. Once the doctor had finished manipulating the man's limbs, he stood back placed his thumb and forefinger on his jaw, canted his head slightly, and looked at his work. After a few seconds he smiled and seemed to approve of everything he had done, and gave orders to have the man taken to x-ray to have pictures taken of the injured parts. At that point, the thought occurred to me that the orthopedic doctor was reasonably sure that we were dealing with dislocated joints rather than actual fractures, and that may have been why he took off his lab coat and unbuttoned and rolled up his sleeves before pulling on the misshapen limbs. It looked as though most of his concern was to see through the x-rays if any real damage had been done to the pelvis of the patient who incidentally was lightly sedated before the manipulation began. To see a transformation like that in the matter of 15 to 30 seconds, to me, was astounding and spoke to the talent of that doctor who was called to the emergency room to do his work.

WATER, WATER, EVERYWHERE

Going through my mind was the thought of me tumbling over the side when the sled dropped that eight inches.

In Center City Philadelphia there is always a construction project large or small going on at any given time. In this case a building was being erected about seven or eight stories tall, and it was just a concrete open framework at this stage. There were no walls or windows in place. We were directed to the fifth floor of this open structure, to attend to a man who had collapsed to the floor while working. When we came upon the scene, we found a construction worker lying on the floor who had obviously had a cardiac event take place while working. We began to work on him, but things did not look very good since some time had elapsed before we had gotten to the scene. There was no elevator in place and we had to hump the equipment up the five flights of stairs to the correct floor. As we worked on him, we were able to visualize a very fine v-fib (ventricular fibrillation) that had to be moved into a coarse v-fib in order to shock the patient. After the administration of several medications the monitor showed us a rhythm that we thought had a chance of converting with a shock, so we charged the monitor immediately. I placed the paddles on the patient's chest in the appropriate positions, and tripped the triggers. I was immediately thrown backwards about seven or eight feet. I received a shock equal to a kick in the chest. I had not noticed in the excitement, that someone had thrown a bucket of water on the patient before our arrival in an attempt to revive him. In working on the patient, I had moved around, and inadvertently placed my knee into a small puddle on the floor, which in addition to the water on the patient and his clothing had conducted some of the shock to me. Shaking off the shock, and returning to my position, we came to the conclusion that the shock had not produced the desired result. His rhythm had deteriorated to such a point that he was unrecoverable by any means at our disposal. We continue to work on him with CPR and began to set him up for transport to the closest emergency room. It was impossible to carry him down five flights of steps, so the construction crew directed us to a flat sled with low sides suspended from a crane against the fifth floor of the building. They informed me that this sled was used to bring supplies and equipment from the street level up to the fifth floor, and that it was completely safe for us to enter the sled as long as we did not stand up. We had a portable stretcher with us that we slid into the sled, placed our equipment there, and climbed in with the patient, still continuing CPR. As we swung away from the building I began to visualize newspaper headlines about a patient and rescue squad team being killed in a construction accident. The sides of the sled were only about a foot high, and as I looked around, I noticed that one of the corner turnbuckles was in a position where it could slip and drop the sled about eight inches until it came to its full length. Going through my mind was the thought of me tumbling over the side when the sled dropped that eight inches and I lost my balance, being on one knee in the sled. Considerably unnerving was the fact that when the four construction workers pushed the sled away from the building it began to sway back and forth in midair as it descended to the ground slowly, giving me another reason to be uneasy about my predicament. As the swaying diminished, I could see we were getting closer to the ground, and at about eight feet from landing, my worst fears were realized, when the turnbuckle slipped and dropped the corner of the sled eight inches. There were many verbal exclamations from the other people riding in the sled with us when this happened, and I think we were all very glad when we touched the ground and the patient was removed to the rescue squad. To this day when I see a construction site I always think of the ride I had, courtesy of the crane operator in Center City. Despite all the hard work to try to recover the patient, none of our efforts were successful and he was pronounced dead in the emergency room. We found with time and experience, that if we could not recover them on the street where they lay, their chances of being recovered in an emergency room were very marginal. I have seen the emergency rooms recover people that we were unable to resuscitate, but I've never seen one leave the hospital and return to a normal life.

NO SMEARED LIPSTICK

We were called to finalize what everyone already knew.

Sometimes people call for a rescue squad even when it is obvious to everyone present, that we will be unable to do anything for the patient. Many accidents involve such severe damage to the patient that even to the untrained eye it is obvious that they are beyond help from anyone. This short story is just such an instance where we were called north of the station in an area of mixed usage. There are streets of row homes interspersed with commercial and industrial buildings. When you have a mixed usage area such as this one, there is a mix of traffic, which includes medium and large trucks. Pedestrians have to be doubly careful when crossing streets, and should not wait for traffic signals to change by standing off the curb in the street. This case is about an elderly woman, obviously in her eighties, dressed completely in an outfit from about 1950. She had on the black tie shoes with a short fat heel, opaque flesh colored stockings, an imitation lambswool coat, a scarf and a hat with a veil in black. She was waiting for the light to change about three steps from the curb in the crosswalk, when a tractor-trailer turned left onto the street she was going to walk across. As we all know, in order for a tractor-trailer to enter a narrower street, they must drive straight ahead as far as they can and then begin the turn into the street, so the rear of the trailer will not scrape vehicles parked on the left side. The woman obviously wasn't paying attention to the tractor-trailer, and when the cab went past her she took a step out into the street and was caught by the rear wheels of the trailer and was knocked down. As she fell she rolled face up and landed in the street just as the rear wheels reached her and rolled over her head. When I arrived, there was a small crowd gathered on the sidewalk, and the tractor-trailer had stopped two feet past her body, which was still lying in the street. I approached to see what her condition was and if there was anything we could do to help her. There was not. The remarkable thing that struck me immediately was that even though her head was crushed there was no blood, and the trauma of the accident did not even smear her lipstick, which I had a problem reconciling in my head. It was just a case where she was beyond help from the moment of impact, and just like putting a dot at the end of the sentence we were called to finalize what everyone already knew. We left her where she was, because a police van was already on location and they would transport her to the morgue. All fatal traffic accidents were investigated by the police department. We went back into service.

TOYS

*The officer was in a panic, soaked with sweat,
and obviously at the end of his wits.*

North of Market Street there is a Hispanic community, and this is where we were directed. It would prove to be an interesting case in every way, starting with us pulling up in front of the assigned address. Out in front of the building I saw a sight that you would never see in the city of Philadelphia, a police car parked at an angle toward the curb with the door open, motor running, and lights revolving. For a police officer to leave his car that fast, I knew that there was something drastically wrong about this scenario, and I was right. We were in front of the typical Philadelphia brownstone converted to apartments. I gathered my equipment and entered the dwelling where I heard talk upstairs, so I mounted the stairs two at a time. I came upon a group of Hispanics on the first floor landing, and another group further up on the next landing. They were gathered around a doorway to an apartment, and parted to let me enter. In the middle of the room was the officer with a small boy face down, draped across a kitchen chair. The officer was attempting some sort of rudimentary artificial respiration, the type that used to be used on a beach to revive a drowned person. He was pressing and releasing on the child's back, and it seemed he was having little or no effect because the child was a bright shade of blue. The officer was in a panic, soaked with sweat, and obviously at the end of his wits when I arrived. When he looked up and saw me come through the door, he looked like someone who had just been told that he had won the lottery. I understood immediately that there was a respiratory issue going on, and removed the child from the chair and placed him on the floor. I turned on the oxygen bottles, and applied the mask to his face and pressed the valve. I fully expected him to respond with a nice rise in his chest, because I had an excellent position to ventilate him. To my surprise, the equipment was unable to penetrate into his lungs. There was an obstruction. I looked into the mouth and could see no obstruction, so I tried again, to no avail. I was unable to get the type of ventilation that I usually got, and was now faced with a very big problem. I felt for a pulse, and the child had a bounding pulse hammering away in his little blue body, and he was destined to stay that way unless I could ferret out the reason why I could not ventilate him. I identified the mother of the child, who was in the kitchen nearby, and asked her what he had been doing before he became ill. She reported that he was playing with a toy car in the kitchen near her. I asked her to bring me the toy, which she produced very quickly. I saw that a wheel was missing from the toy, and asked the mother if it had had all four wheels when her son was playing with it. She said that he was rolling the truck around on the floor and it had four wheels, so I knew where the missing wheel had gone. The wheel was stuck in the child's airway, and I was ventilating through the axel hole in the rubber wheel. I removed the oxygen mask and rolled the child back and forth on the linoleum floor trying to get a better airway. I again attempted to force oxygen past the wheel, with slightly better success. He started to slowly turn less blue, and was showing areas of pink to his skin. I stopped ventilating him again and picked him up upside down and pumped him rapidly up and down, holding him by his ankles. When I placed him down this time I had opened the airway enough to get some normal color, so I called that a win, and made the decision that he was stable enough to get him outside, and into the rescue for the trip to Children's Hospital. My partner Ken Gary had used his time effectively in soliciting help to get the stretcher brought up to the room, and the child was placed onto it. We carried him out and placed him into the squad, continuing the forced ventilation, as his eyelids began to flicker. He was waking up. We placed a call to the hospital reporting the child's predicament, so they were ready for our arrival. Later, he was taken to the operating room, and the wheel was removed from his trachea. I don't think the police officer had much stamina to finish his shift, after what he had just been through. I'll also bet he took a class in CPR at his first opportunity.

THE SPIRAL STAIRCASE

There was no way this woman would survive
a trip up the spiral staircase to the street.

Saturday night in any fire station is usually a busy time, and I, like all young men, preferred to work on shifts where exciting things were bound to happen. The fire rescue service was no exception to this rule and many, many, exciting things happened on Friday and Saturday nights in Center City. People would go out on the town after working all week, and many of the Center City attractions were full of people enjoying themselves. To draw in some of the people looking for food and drink, there is a myriad of bars and restaurants on the side streets, each with its own ambience. On this particular Saturday night we were dispatched to one of these bars on a side street, which was located in the basement of a building. When you walked in the front door you were confronted with a metal spiral staircase going down one level to a large nightclub with a bar in the center of the room. We carried all of our equipment down the spiral staircase, leaving the stretcher in the rescue squad, because there was no way it would fit down the stairway in front of us. As we reached the bottom of the staircase, we were directed around to the far side of the bar where a young black woman was lying on the floor near an overturned barstool. She appeared to be in her twenties and very well dressed. She was accompanied by her date and several other couples who stood around her. A quick examination showed that she was not breathing, so I started CPR and ventilated her while my partner placed her on the heart monitor for a quick look.

Immediately we saw that she was in ventricular fibrillation, and charged the monitor as we placed the paddles on her chest. I delivered a shock as soon as the monitor showed it was ready. She went flat line which was usual, and came back with another run of ventricular fibrillation as we continued the CPR on her. She did not convert. It was necessary to immediately start an IV and administer medication starting with an amp of lidocaine. I had just had a conversation with one of our supervising physicians about how to get a patient out of ventricular fibrillation when shocking had no effect. His advice was that you had to reduce the irritability of the heart so that after the shock was administered, only one focus would be left to start the heartbeat again. In ventricular fibrillation multiple areas in the heart are all firing at the same time, giving the fibrillating rhythm. Remembering the physician's explanation, I decided to continue to administer lidocaine until she converted. The monitor was charged, and the second shock was delivered into her chest, and it too was unsuccessful. I felt that we had no other option but to use another lidocaine injection since our protocol was maxed out with the two doses we had given. I had just used my last amp of lidocaine, so I placed a call for another rescue squad to come to the scene to provide additional needed medications. The patient still showed a coarse ventricular fibrillation, and our CPR was doing a good job of making a pulse with each thrust on her chest. When the second rescue squad arrived several minutes later, I requested an amp of lidocaine from them, and administered it immediately to the patient. I understood that there was no way this young woman would survive a trip up the spiral staircase to the street, because there was no way to continue to ventilate her and do CPR in a stair chair. A stair chair was the only appliance we had access to that could be used to carry a patient up a spiral staircase to the street level. I knew that we had to restore a pulse and blood pressure where she lay, because she would never make it as a viable patient to the emergency room if we had to go up the stairs. This thought went through my mind, as I pushed the last amp of lidocaine into her, and charged the monitor for a third time. I was hoping that this amp would do the trick, and anesthetize her enough to get a good conversion. My partner placed the paddles on her, and yelled, "Clear!", as I took my hands from her body. She jumped from the shock delivered into her chest. My eyes were glued onto the monitor screen, as a flat line progressed from the left to right, waiting for her heart to respond after the shock. After what seemed like an eternity, the monitor showed a good solid beat on the screen, followed by another, and then a nice normal sinus rhythm. Continuing to breathe for her, I immediately felt for a pulse on her neck, and it was present. At that point we decided to make arrangements to place her into a stair chair, and applied the straps to her chest to get ready to move her to the stairway. We took a blood pressure, which showed an acceptable reading, and as we did this, she took her first spontaneous breath. This was an added plus, because it gave me the opportunity to place a nasal cannula with a long lead to get her up to the street. Since the second rescue squad was present, we had ample help to assist in moving her up the spiral staircase, allowing two men to go up backward at the head, and one facing forward at the feet. She was taken to the closest emergency room where we were later told she indeed had had a heart attack. We were informed that she was placed into cardiac care, and was sitting up talking the next day, like nothing had happened. She had absolutely no idea how lucky she had been on that Saturday night.

There was a second exit from the basement, but it was in the rear of the building leading to two metal doors in the pavement through which kegs of beer were delivered.

DENT IN THE DOOR

*When I looked up I could see a light coming from
an open window very high up on the building.*

The theater district in Philadelphia has many restaurants, and all have an area on a rear street where they take deliveries and put out the garbage. During the day no parking is allowed on the streets because of the many deliveries of provisions that are supplied to these establishments by large trucks. In the evening however, parking is allowed, and many theatergoers hunt for free parking places on these back streets. On this evening it had just finished raining, and the streets were wet as the show let out. The streets in every direction around the theater had people in them going to their parked cars. In this case, we got a call to go to one of the back streets because one of these couples had made an almost fatal discovery. As they were walking on the sidewalk toward their car the body of a woman wearing a blue nightgown and a full length fur coat crashed to the ground not two feet in front of them. When we arrived, the woman was hysterical and her companion was trying to calm her down. They had almost been struck by the falling woman. She had hit the ground so hard that it had broken her head open, and her brains had traveled toward the street with such force that it dented the door of a pickup truck parked at the curb. There was a large bloody fluid mark in the center of the door where the brains had hit, and they continued to slide down the door and were resting in the gutter in a pile. When I looked up I could see the light coming from an open window very high up on the building and curtains blowing out into the night. Obviously, she had launched herself out of the window without looking below to see if she would endanger anyone on the street. When the police arrived they went up inside the building to the floor with the open window, and gained entry to the apartment. They discovered that the woman lived alone, and she had been sitting in a chair in the middle of the room facing the open window. The chair had been placed in that position by the woman earlier in the night, and she had sat facing the window for a long time. A stool was placed up against the radiator in the room to be used as a stepping stone to launch from the window. She must have gotten cold from the evening air coming in the open window, so she went into the closet leaving the door open and retrieved the fur coat which she put on over her blue nightgown. At the appropriate time for her, she advanced forward stepping on the stool, stepping on the radiator, and dove forward out of the window. The police who had arrived after us, took charge of the scene, and began their investigation starting with the young couple on the street that were almost killed by the falling body. We made ourselves available by radio and returned to our fire station ready for the next call.

I LIED

To our surprise, in a couple minutes, he
woke up as though he had been asleep.

If you left the front door of our fire station, turned left, and drove to the corner you would reach 22nd Street. If you then went a half a block to 22nd and Chestnut you would find a bar on the corner. It was probably less than a minute from the firehouse. On this day about 5:30 in the afternoon we received a call to respond to this bar. Upon arrival we parked on 22nd Street. I grabbed the oxygen and the drug box and went in the ladies' entrance to the bar. There on the floor was an overturned barstool and a man, who had slow gasping type respirations, lying on the floor. I examined him quickly, and found that he had no pulse, and his breathing was in the process of shutting down from lack of oxygen to the breathing centers in the brain. I immediately began CPR, ventilating with 100% pure oxygen as I waited for my partner to arrive with the heart monitor/ defibrillator. As the CPR progressed, the man's respirations returned to what seemed like normal, once the chest compressions had begun. His eyelids began to flicker, and I got the impression he was returning to consciousness with just CPR. I stopped for a minute thinking that he may have had a pulse that I just could not feel, and I was doing compressions for nothing. As soon as I stopped, everything began to return as it was when I found him, so I started again. After another short burst of oxygen and CPR, again, I received the same impression that he was waking up. At that time my partner came in with the monitor and defibrillator and I asked him to please place the patient on the monitor quickly and charge the defibrillator. We used the wire leads to hook him to the monitor because it was faster than trying to cut through two shirts, and a thick sweater. The monitor showed a coarse ventricular fibrillation, so we cut through his clothes after all. As soon as we got his chest clear, we applied the gel and delivered a shock announced by a large thump. Just before the shock we had started running a tape to verify the v-fib, and his conversion, if it happened. After a few seconds the flat line disappeared, and a normal sinus rhythm showed on the monitor. Since we were hardwired to the patient and the tape was clean, there could be no doubt that he had been converted by us. We started an IV, and pushed an amp of lidocaine to prevent a reoccurrence of the v-fib before we got him to the hospital. To our surprise, in a couple minutes, he woke up as though he had been asleep, ripped out the IV, and announced he was getting up and going home from the bar. At this time I put my hand on his chest to keep him from rising, and explained to him that he had been dead on the floor. He looked to the bartender for verification. He seemed to know the bartender very well, and the bartender confirmed what I had said. Further to our conversation I announced that I given him a medication through the IV and when it wore off he was likely to die if we did not get him to the emergency room quickly. Of course that was a lie, but there was a likelihood that he could have another episode at any time, without professional medical care. He looked again to the bartender, asking him if what I said was true, and the bartender replied that he had seen us give him a medication, and what I said might be true. With that, the man on the floor agreed to let us take him to the University of Pennsylvania Medical Center emergency room, which was just across the bridge from where we were. We applied a bandage to his arm, because he was bleeding from the open vein, and wasted no time in placing him on the stretcher and removing him from the bar. We called ahead to let them know what we had, and that we had had a problem getting consent from the man to be treated. We had received information from the bartender that the patient had fallen off the stool, appeared to be unconscious, and laid on the floor for a moment. Just as the bartender was going around the bar to assist the man, he got up from the floor set the barstool up right, and climbed back on it. After several more minutes he had again passed out, fell to the floor, and the same action was repeated the second time. On the third fall from the stool, the patient did not get up, and 911 was called, and we responded. This information tells me that he had suffered an unknown arrhythmia which rendered him unconscious, but was not fatal. Fortunate for him it had repaired itself twice, keeping him at the bar, until he had the third attack. Had he left the bar and made it to his home down the street, he would have suffered a fatal attack at home and would not have survived since he lived alone. For some reason unknown to me, people in bars seem to be the luckiest individuals in society.

ELECTRIC TRAIN

We only carried two vials of morphine,
and he got both of them.

Going left and down the street from the firehouse, loomed a very large, gray building called 30th Street, Station. It was quite a large train station built around the turn of the century, and was still in heavy use. We were sent along with an engine company, a ladder company, and battalion chief to deal with a problem on an unused train platform in the lower levels of the station. We were met at the door to the main entrance on Market Street by train personnel who guided us through the maze of stairs and platforms to the appropriate area. We carried all of our equipment and stretcher down two flights of steps to a lower level which appeared dark and unused. As we rolled the stretcher along with all the equipment we were directed to a center platform that had an unused darkened train parked alongside it. This section of the train station was used to park extra train cars during off peak hours. All of the cars were electric and had large pantographs extending upward from the top of the train to the charged electrical wire overhead. Everything on the platform was dark, so the only light in the area was from equipment carried by the firemen. We were shown down the center of the platform where the trainman directed us to look on the top of one of the electric cars. Up on the roof writhing in pain was a young black male covered in char from severe burns. Luckily the ladder company present, had brought with them a short ladder, in case it was needed. I used this ladder to climb up near the man, after being assured that no electrical lines were alive where we were working. I asked the engine company and ladder company to assist me in bringing the burned man down from the top of the train so he could be treated. I grabbed his arm, and pulled him toward the edge of the train where others could get a hand on him as he slid down from the top of the car. When I let go of his wrist a handful of burned flesh remained in the palm of my hand. He was placed on the stretcher, but considering the amount of pain he was experiencing, he was not lying still. I immediately reached into the drug box, withdrew a Tubex, inserted a preload of morphine, and injected him directly into a vein in the antecubital area. I thought that considering the amount of pain he was experiencing there would be no harm in giving him a direct injection of morphine to try to get him under control. I made the assumption that both his blood pressure and pulse were elevated, and his respirations were certainly adequate enough to tolerate the drug. We took a moment to do a quick assessment as he began to calm down enough for us to get an IV started. We hung a large bag of IV fluid through which we pushed another Tubex of morphine. (We only carried two vials of morphine and he got both of them.) Once the morphine entered his system he began to settle down enough for us to move him from the area without fear of him tossing and turning and throwing himself off the stretcher onto the floor. We transported him to the University of Pennsylvania emergency room where he was stabilized, and later moved to the Chester Crozier Burn Unit. Several days later, his story was published in the local paper and elaborated upon by a police officer who stopped into the firehouse to grab a snack.

He told us that the young man had approached a contact in the train station to conclude a homosexual tryst. They sought out an unused section of the station that was appropriate for their needs; however, things were about to change to something unexpected. The second individual pulled a knife in order to conduct an armed robbery of the man who was severely burned. After he had taken the victim's wallet, and wristwatch, he had him undress, and throw his clothes on the top of the train, some of which were draped over both the pantograph and the charged electrical wire above it. The victim dressed in only his under shorts and socks climbed up a fixed ladder on the end of the train car to retrieve his clothing. As he reached up to get his clothing he grabbed the electrical wire to steady himself, and received a full charge of electricity used to power the trains. This sudden surge in power tripped all of the circuit breakers in that section of the station, bringing train personnel to the platform to look for the cause of the outage. It was then, that they discovered the burned young man on the top of the car and radioed for fire rescue immediately. The article in the newspaper was followed 10 days later by a notice that he had died of his injuries while being treated in the burn center. The thief was never found.

WHY?

She had sustained third degree burns over most of her body, and she lay in the street shivering from shock.

Many times the police get to a location before the fire rescue squad, and sometimes they remove the patient to a hospital before the rescue squad gets on the scene. In this story the police had indeed arrived at the scene before us, and took three burn cases to the hospital before we arrived. The case that they left for us, was of course, the most serious, and it was obvious why they did not want to touch her. The story we received from the patient, who was a young girl in her teens, burned over 90% of her body is recounted below.

We found her lying on the ground about 10 feet away from a burning car, surrounded by onlookers who had no idea how to help her. The girl and her boyfriend were in the backseat of a two-door car, with two other boys in the front. The car had stopped out from the curb, to talk to others who had been walking up the street, and who were then leaning in the window of the car. As they all conversed, another car full of young men approached, and pulled up close to the stopped vehicle. With vehicles lined up side-by-side, a container filled with gasoline was thrown into the window of the first car. Since those inside were all smoking cigarettes, it burst into flame, and caused an immediate panic. The car with the young men sped off, and left the others to their fate, which was to suffer serious burns to their bodies in varying degrees, as the car began to incinerate. Those in the front seat of the vehicle jumped out immediately through the front doors, and set about tearing off those articles of clothing that were on fire. The boy and girl in the back seat of the car were faced with a bigger problem once those in the front had exited. The problem developed because in this two-door car, people in the back seat could only exit the vehicle one at a time because, the front seat back rests folded inward on each other, effectively preventing the second person from exiting on his side until the first had done so. Or, in this case the boy in the back of the car was faster than the girl, and folded his seat in front of the girl's, allowing him to exit first, and forcing her to follow him out of his side of the car. She was the last person to exit the vehicle, remaining in the searing heat until all the occupants had escaped before her. By that time, she had sustained third-degree burns over almost all of her body, and she lay in the street shivering from shock as body fluids spilled from her body onto the street, leaving a wet outline on the asphalt. We immediately removed her from the pavement and placed her on our stretcher, covering her burned body with a sheet and placed her in the back of the rescue squad. I immediately started two large bore IVs, one in each arm, and hung a couple 1000cc bags of IV fluid to begin replacing all the fluid she was losing. I thought it best to take her immediately to the closest hospital emergency room so she could be stabilized and prepared for shipment to one of the two available burn centers. We arrived at St. Joseph's Hospital emergency room after notifying them that we were en route with a burn victim. They were stunned when they saw the girl we had wheeled in on our stretcher, and I immediately began to get the feeling that we should have just headed for the burn center instead of going to St. Joseph's. Before I left her in the emergency room, she kept repeating over and over through her chattering teeth, that she couldn't understand why someone would want to do that to her, and what did she do to deserve this. As I later found out, her old boyfriend was upset with her for breaking up with him, and had been driving around with his buddies looking for her that afternoon. When he found her in the backseat of the car with her new boyfriend, he threw the gasoline on them both.

I still remember the doctor's eyes as big as saucers and looking stunned, when he pulled back the sheet on the girl, and the nurse covering her face and turning away from the shocking sight of a young girl with all her flesh burned off. Several hours later we heard a call come through for another unit to transfer the girl from St. Joseph's Hospital to Chester Crozier Burn Center, which was the premier burn center serving Philadelphia and the surrounding area, and well outside the city limits. The others present in the car all received burns, but due to her long exposure in the vehicle, she was by far the most seriously burned, and required the most serious and determined interventions from the burn unit staff. I was never able to learn what eventually happened to this young woman.

BAG OF WATERS

*The baby's feet were still inside the mother and
the baby was still inside the bag of liquid.*

Every once in a while the fire rescue unit is called upon
to deliver, or assist in delivering a baby, and this is one
such case. It is remarkable, because it was only one city
block away from the hospital, but the mother did not
have time to negotiate that one city block. This was again
another brownstone multiple occupancy dwelling, where
Ken Gary and I entered the first floor front apartment to
find a woman in bed who was in the process of delivering
a baby in a very odd situation. The baby's feet were still
inside the mother and the baby was completely contained
in this membrane filled with liquid which I assumed was
the bag of waters. Usually, this bag was broken before the
baby was delivered in the normal birth, but this time the
baby was still inside the bag of liquid, and was completely
blue in color. Ken produced a small knife and stuck the
bag of waters with it, and the bag completely disintegrated
spilling the fluid all over the bed. I turned on the oxygen,
and after clearing the baby's airway, began to very gently
administer 100% oxygen to the baby. This had the immediate effect of turning the baby pink, and the baby started
to cry, while still attached to the mother with the umbilical
cord protruding from her vagina. We had a small packet in
our medical box for use in delivering a newborn outside
of the hospital. We tore open the blister pack, and inside
found two umbilical cord clamps, which were applied
close together on the cord, and snapped into place. In the
pack was a small pair of sterile scissors, which was used

to sever the cord, effectively separating the baby from the placenta. Since the baby had a good airway, and was breathing quite well, the next issue to be addressed was keeping the baby warm, so we carefully wrapped it in a hospital blanket and gave it to the mother to hold. There was one other woman in the room who was a friend of the mother, and was attending to her as best she could before we arrived on the scene. We gathered the mother up, placed her on our stretcher, and immediately removed her to the Hahnemann Hospital emergency room where she could complete the delivery under a doctor's care, and the baby could be examined thoroughly. This was a very first time I had ever seen a baby delivered inside the bag of waters. I don't imagine many doctors have seen it either. I later learned that the baby was doing well but had exhibited signs of a Trisomy 21, well known as Down Syndrome.

DON'T BUG ME

The young boy began to thrash around and scream as the beetle tried to scrape its way further inside his head.

This is just a short story about a mother who brought her son, about eight years old, into the firehouse to see the paramedics. The son was acting very peculiar by twitching his head every few seconds, and squinting and blinking with each twitch. Upon questioning the mother, I found that the son had been playing with a small beetle letting it crawl round on his arm while he watched it. About 15 minutes later he came into the house with these symptoms and reported that the beetle was stuck in his ear. The mother took a look and confirmed that there was a dark object deep inside the ear canal, so she brought him over to the firehouse to see what could be done. Since we did not have a scope for examining the ear canal, the best I could do was to shine a flashlight in and spot what appeared to be the beetle inside the canal. Since we did not have the tools for working in an ear canal, a decision was made to take the boy and his mother to the local hospital to be examined by an ear, nose, and throat doctor. After our arrival to Holy Redeemer emergency room, we decided to stay for a short time to assist the doctor in positioning the boy for both examination and removal of the insect. The boy was laid on his side with a pillow under his head with the affected ear facing up toward a bright light. The doctor produced a long thin set of forceps and reached into the ear to grab the beetle and pull it out. When the forceps were extracted the doctor had pinched off a piece of the beetle's abdomen which had the effect of driving the beetle wild in an attempt to claw its way further inside the canal to avoid further injury. The young boy began to thrash around and scream as the beetle tried to scrape its way further inside his head. Understanding that his first attempt at removing the beetle was a failure, the doctor decided to drop a small amount of lidocaine into the ear to anesthetize the tissues that the beetle was irritating. The beetle did not like this tactic either and again forcibly tried to scratch its way into the eardrum. At this point the young boy found it impossible to lie still and got up from the table and started banging the heel of his hand on the opposite side of his head as if to force a water bubble out of his ear. The doctor decided that the only solution at this point was to anesthetize the boy so work could begin in earnest to extract the beetle quickly. The boy received a small dose of anesthesia, and quickly passed out on the table, which allowed the physician to again enter the ear with the forceps and pick the bug apart in pieces effectively killing the bug and removing the sections piecemeal. A series of antiseptic flushes were then squirted into the ear removing an assortment of legs and other chunks and acting as a prevention against an ear infection. The flushes were followed by a shot of penicillin in the behind which completed the treatment. Since the boy and his mother lived around the corner from the firehouse, we loaded them back in the rescue squad, and drove them back to the station so they could walk home. The same boy had been to the firehouse a year before with a penny stuck in his nose that later had to be removed from his sinus cavity during a long procedure in the operating room of the local hospital.

THE TIP

*Foaming liquid kept pouring out of her mouth
with each exhale. Things did not look good.*

Just west of the firehouse across the Market Street Bridge
is the campus of the University of Pennsylvania. And just
north of the campus is a section of mixed housing where
an eclectic group of black people live. In this section are
older people that have lived in the homes for years, and
interspersed throughout this community are groups of young
militant blacks who seemed to get into a significant amount
of trouble with the law, and sooner or later they all wound
up in the emergency room of the local hospital. This is a
story of three such cases from that community. In the first
case Ken Gary and I responded to a home occupied by an
older black lady who was in the second floor rear bedroom,
suffering from a severe case of pulmonary edema. Upon our
arrival she was sitting in a chair partially leaning out of an
open window gasping for breath. After a quick listen with a
stethoscope I determined that her lungs were filled with fluid
and she was trying to breathe through the liquid. Her flesh
was ashen in color, she was soaked in sweat, and breathing
was very laborious. She had obviously been in that condition for an extended period of time as she was completely
exhausted and at the point of collapse, which she did a few
minutes after our arrival. She fell from the chair to the floor
and we immediately went to work on her try to keep her
alive. Ken began to administer 100% oxygen to her while I
quickly started an IV with a microdripper and administered
a dose of Lasix through the pinched off tubing. (A microdripper is used to prevent the IV fluid being administered

too quickly and overwhelming an already compromised system.) Ken was having trouble ventilating her because foaming liquid kept pouring out of her mouth with each exhale. Things did not look good as I attempted to get a blood pressure. Unable to hear a blood pressure and unable to feel the pulse, I began CPR hoping I could circulate enough Lasix through her system to draw down the edema enough for her to breathe. After several long minutes of performing CPR, I felt for a pulse, which I was able to find in her neck, so I again attempted to gain a blood pressure which registered at 70 over zero. Ken also found he was able to ventilate the lady much easier because the fluid level in her lung was definitely decreasing to a manageable level. It was at this point that we decided to transfer her to the hospital before another issue developed that would complicate things. It's important to remember that we were dealing with a patient of advanced age which may have had other underlying problems. Ken went to get the equipment we would need to move her and encountered several young men waiting downstairs who he enlisted to help. They were very eager to help the relative get to the hospital and were stunned when they saw that she was unconscious lying on the floor, because last time they saw her she was sitting in a chair leaning out the window. They made an assumption that we had caused her to become unconscious, and began to raise their voices about the quality of care that she was receiving. I quickly informed them that I wouldn't have treated my own mother any differently, and I was doing the best that could be done for her under the circumstances. That seemed to calm them down, and they were a great help in removing her from the second floor and placing her in the rescue squad. We removed her to Presbyterian Hospital and placed her in the emergency room where the staff took over her care. We made ourselves available after restoring all our equipment and changing the oxygen bottles. We returned to the station not anticipating that we would hear anything further about this case.

About a month later, Ken and I were called to the deputy

chief's office where he had some information to give us about the patient we had administered to on that particular day. He informed Ken and I that the woman whom we had treated wanted to meet with us and give us some money. Instinctively, both Ken and I voiced opposition to receiving money from anyone for our services, although we did not mind seeing the woman again alive and healthy. I was stunned when the deputy chief told us that we would take the rescue squad and go to this meeting, and if the woman handed us an envelope with money in it we were to accept it and to thank her profusely for the gift. I was sort of stunned with that order, and felt embarrassed to go to a meeting where we would receive anything of value and be ordered to take it. As ordered, we went back to the lady's home. As we entered the front door we encountered a group of people seated in the living room. I looked around at everyone there, but was unable to recognize our patient under these circumstances. A woman stood up and walked over to us and introduced herself as the woman whose name I had typed on the report. She wanted to shake hands with each of us and in the process presented each of us with a white envelope and voiced how appreciative she was for the work we had done. Both Ken and I were extremely embarrassed, but we were able to voice how happy we were that treating her was so successful, because she currently looked a picture of health and happiness and we were stunned how different she looked from the night we had worked on her. After answering a few questions from the group and expressing our thanks for the kind remarks, Ken and I went back on duty and left the home. When we opened our envelopes each of us received $50 from the woman, which I'm sure represented a significant portion of her income for the month. I thought over and over how much of a sacrifice it must have been for that woman to share her meager income with us for a job well done. It was the first and only time either Ken or I had ever received any thanks for our work.

OD

*We watched as the medication did an
excellent job of defeating the narcotic.*

This case was about two blocks away from where we
had treated the lady with pulmonary edema. It was very
close to the hospital emergency room, only about 300 yards
away. We had received a call when we were already on the
road, about eight to nine blocks away from the address.
Our arrival on the scene was very quick. We brought our
usual equipment to the front door of the home which was
already ajar. As we entered, we encountered a young man
who appeared to be in his twenties lying flat on the floor
face up with no respirations visible. As I knelt beside him
I immediately went for a pulse on the neck. It was there,
so we began to administer oxygen forcing it into his lungs
with each press of the mouthpiece. A quick blood pressure
revealed that the man was hypotensive. Several subse-
quent blood pressures revealed that he was stabilizing to
a normal pressure after being treated. Examination of his
pupils revealed that they were pinpoint, and they were
unreactive to light. My initial thoughts were that he had
either ingested or injected a drug into his system which had
caused respiratory arrest after a brief period of time. Since
we carried a medication called Narcan to be used in just
this instance, I drew up and injected a dose of this medication into our newly placed IV line. It had the property
of sitting on the same receptor sites as heroin derivatives
and counteracting their effects rather quickly. I continued
to monitor him taking both pulse and blood pressure and
recording the numbers as Ken continued to ventilate. We

watched as the medication did an excellent job of defeating the narcotic. We began to see signs of the patient improving. His respirations began to return to normal, so we were able to support him with just the oxygen instead of breathing for him. We picked him up, placed him on our stretcher, and took him to the Presbyterian Hospital emergency room, where he returned to consciousness on their stretcher. After explaining to the doctor what we had done, it was interesting to continue to observe this patient as he immediately went into drug withdrawal suffering from a case of DTs right there on the table. As he became fully conscious of his surroundings, he started rubbing his arms and stating, "I got to get cool," over and over again. The doctor tried to explain to him how close he had come to death lying in that entryway of the house, but he wasn't interested. He just continued to repeat, "I got to get cool." I assumed that meant that he wanted another dose of narcotic which he wasn't going to get in that hospital. Both Ken and I felt that we had wasted our time and our efforts in treating this young man, whom we felt was destined for a very short life.

WRONG

*He instructed the nurse to write down our names
from our nametags, because he was going to
write a letter to the fire department to reprimand
us for our wrong treatment of the patient.*

Even doctors make mistakes. This is a story about one
such incident concerning the same neighborhood, the
same hospital, and the same emergency room. It was an
early morning call in the early spring, at a time when all
the trees are just beginning to put out their new leaves, and
yellow pollen is dusting every flat surface. It was another
case of a man sitting in the back bedroom on a chair by
the window attempting to get more air into his respiratory
system which was rapidly closing off. He was drenched in
sweat, and was having severe difficulty inhaling, and was
in a panic for air. A quick listen to his lungs told me that
he had a constriction in his airway, probably brought on by
asthma or allergies. Since we carried a medication called
epinephrine which in the correct dose would treat this problem, it was quickly administered subcutaneously, as called
for in our protocol. Since this medication is administered
under the skin it takes a while to take effect, so the object
is to keep the patient calm, assist them with their breathing
as much as possible, and wait until the medication takes
effect. Usually, in these cases the patients cannot tolerate a
mask over their faces since it gives them a claustrophobic
feeling, even though there is oxygen flowing through it in a
large volume. In this case we had to be satisfied with placing a nasal cannula, and making preparations to remove the
patient to the emergency room. Having the patient move as

little as possible is a key feature, because the object is to
have the patient expend as little oxygen as necessary until
the medication opens the airways further. We were able to
get the patient into the rescue squad without much effort,
and took him to the emergency room where I gave the report
to the attending doctor. When I explained my course of
treatment he immediately flew off the handle, and accused
me of harming the patient by giving the wrong medication,
and further stated that I was lucky that my misdiagnosis
didn't kill the patient while en route to the hospital. He
further stated that these are the kind of things that happen
when you take a bunch of firemen off the street, and let
them ride around giving medications to people unsuper-
vised. He instructed the nurse to write down our names
from our nametags, because he was going to write a letter
to the fire department to reprimand us for our wrong treatment of this patient. All this happened before he had examined the patient, or took a listen to the patient's lungs. He
was so sure that he knew what was wrong as soon as he
saw the patient sitting on the stretcher laboring to breathe.
He went into the cubicle to do his thing, and had the nurse
draw a syringe full of Lasix to be given to the man because
he was sure that the patient was in pulmonary edema and
not suffering from a constricted airway that I had treated.
The nurse went about her job preparing a syringe and the
doctor continued to berate me in the emergency room while
he waited to administer the medication. He seemed so full
of anger that something in the past must have caused him
to act this way. As the nurse presented him with a syringe
the patient spoke in a very loud voice, "Whew, I thought I
was a goner there for a few minutes! Oh my God, I feel so
much better now. That was rough!" Upon hearing this the
doctor put down the Lasix syringe and walked away. The
medication I had given had finally taken full effect and
relieved the patient's symptoms. I had been vindicated just
in time, and it wasn't necessary to inject the patient with
an overwhelming dose of a medication he did not need to

receive. The doctor realized he was wrong, but just walked away and busied himself with something in another room so he did not have to look me in the eye again, especially since he had made so many negative comments. Before I left the emergency room I asked the nurse who had drawn up the medication if she thought that the doctor would like more information on my name and the rescue unit so he could complete his letter to the fire department. She told me that she was sure he had more than enough. If he wrote a letter about me I never heard anything about it and neither did Ken.

MY NOSE, MY NOSE

*We found out later that the man was admitted to
the hospital and never did return home again.*

Anyone working the rescue squad, sooner or later has a
patient that is chronically ill, and calls for service repeatedly day after day after day after day. This was one of
those cases of the sickly old man who lived his life in bed,
surrounded by pill bottles, and juices and urinals, and all
those things that accumulate around the sickbed. This was
a thin, pale, old man in a darkened bedroom with all the
shades and curtains drawn and a very tall bedside lamp, the
only light on in the room. Though in an expensive building,
and expensively furnished, the place was dark and dingy,
and smelled musty. He was what we called a COPDer, on
oxygen through a nasal cannula, with a very high pitched
nasally voice which had sort of a whiny tone. His wife
was in attendance, and she appeared aged, with long gray
hair drawn up in a bun and fixed in place with bobbie pins
which were partially sticking out of her head. She seemed
very concerned about his condition and continuously
hovered over Ron and me as we administered to the old
man, starting with a set of vital signs, which for his condition were normal. At the bedside there was a lamp on the
table with a very large shade about three feet high, a carafe
of orange juice, several partially filled glasses of liquid,
and a pile of straws. Slid up against the table and touching
the bed was an old tin TV tray, and on the tray was what
looked like a hundred pill bottles all with their lids off.
The old man had reported that he couldn't catch his breath
which prompted Ron to approach close. He was forced to

slide the tray full of pills carefully to the side to have a listen to the man's lungs, by having him lean forward and placing a stethoscope on his back. After a good listen Ron attempted to stand up straight again but the back of his elbow bumped the lampshade causing the lamp to start to fall over. Ron quickly tried to catch it, but not before it struck the carafe of orange juice which launched toward the multitude of open pill containers. Ron seeing disaster approaching, let go of the lamp and attempted to grab the orange juice before it spilled into the open pill containers. He was unable to grab it in time. As the juice flowed out of the large carafe all over the pills, he was struck in the head by the lamp which to his horror crashed down on top of the juice and all the pill containers. The few pills containers that the juice missed, were upset by the crashing lamp onto the tray full if juice. I thought the elderly wife was going to have a heart attack. She had both hands up over her head shaking her fingers and yelling, "No, no, no!" The husband screamed in his high-pitched voice as Ron apologized for causing such a mess. At that point the reason for the call was forgotten. Both Ron and I were thrown unceremoniously out of the apartment by the old lady, as she called Ron "a dumb ass".

About two weeks later on a night shift we were recalled back to the same apartment, and as the door opened, the same old lady was struck with horror as she saw Ron standing in front of me in the hall. She allowed us both to enter the apartment but would not allow Ronald to enter the bedroom. Remembering her prior statement she told Ron to wait by the door as she let me examine the patient. As I entered the bedroom, I was greeted by the same lamp, but with no shade and just a bare light bulb, as the shade was destroyed during our last encounter. The carafe of juice, all the glasses, and straws were in the same position, as was the aluminum tray with all the pill bottles on it, only this time they all had their caps on. The old lady remarked to me that Ron had cost her a fortune in renewing all the prescriptions that had been destroyed by the juice and the lamp. An examination of her husband showed that his condition had deteriorated since our last visit, and the decision was made to remove him to the emergency room. Ron was allowed into the room with the stretcher, only to assist me with getting him on the stretcher, and making him comfortable for the ride to the hospital. We were to take the patient, but the old lady was going to follow in a couple minutes, after putting on some clothing. I placed the old man on oxygen in the rescue squad and Ron drove us to the emergency room. Oxygen in the squad was fed by a large bottle strapped to the wall that we could connect the patient's tubing to. When the doors opened at the hospital, Ron released the stretcher, but in the confusion, I had not unplugged the oxygen tubing from the wall unit. When we rolled the stretcher out, the nasal cannula was still attached from his nose to the wall and unfortunately his nostrils were pulled up towards his eyes, which was momentarily uncomfortable. The old man began to yell about the pain he felt from getting his nose pulled by the tubing. His high-pitched voice was almost comical. I quickly realized my mistake and reattach the cannula to the portable oxygen unit on the stretcher. Through this he began to whine in his high-pitched voice, "My nose, my nose, they tried to rip off my nose!" as we wheeled him through the emergency room doors. He continued to yell, "My nose, my nose!" to the first doctor we reached who began to examine his nose, until we were able to tell him that the gentleman actually had a breathing problem, and there was nothing really wrong with his nose. In short order, we transferred him over to the hospital's equipment, gathered our things together, and Ron and I went back to the firehouse. We found out later that the man was admitted to the hospital that evening and never did return home again.

LUCK RAN OUT

*"You're going to die, you've been shot in the heart.
Why not tell us everything you know before you die."*

This is a story of a very unusual case involving Ivan
Greenstein who lived in an apartment almost next door to
the firehouse on Bustleton Avenue. He rented an apartment
in a large complex and set himself up in business selling
drugs to a local clientele. On this particular day a young
black man had knocked on his door and indicated that he
was conducting an armed robbery with a loaded revolver
and he wanted all of Ivan's money. Realizing that he was
in jeopardy Ivan attempted to close the door on the robber,
but was too slow, because the robber fired a shot into Ivan's
chest. When we arrived on the scene, Ivan was being brought
outside by police. We saw him coming, so we pulled our
stretcher from the rear of the squad and Ivan was placed
on it. To put it mildly, he looked horrible. He was pale as a
ghost, sweating, breathing shallowly, and had a bullet hole
in his chest exactly where his heart would be found underneath his ribs. A small amount of blood ran from the wound
down the front of him and was staining his pants, and he
was bare chested. A police officer was questioning him very
nervously, trying to get some information out of him before
he died on the spot from a bullet in the heart. The officer
stated, "You're going to die, you've been shot in the heart.
Why not tell us everything you know before you die," and
he kept repeating this over and over, even as we loaded him
into the rescue squad. The officer continued probing Ivan
asking him to reveal who shot him, and any other information he could gain. Ivan said nothing. We indicated to the

police that we had to go, and called ahead to the hospital explaining what we had on board, indicating that it appeared that Ivan had a bullet in or around his heart. I placed him on oxygen but made no attempt to dress the wound because the bleeding had stopped. I was totally perplexed because the blood should be squirting from the hole with every beat of his heart. I assessed his lungs and they were mostly clear, and his blood pressure was low but palpable. He remained awake and did not drift off on the ride. As we arrived at the hospital they were waiting for us at the door, and Ivan was quickly taken off our hands. They ran wheeling him inside the hospital, but it was not the last we would hear of Ivan Greenstein. The next day while we were at the hospital emergency room on another case, we asked one of the physicians what the outcome was for Ivan Greenstein. He stated that Ivan was the luckiest guy on the planet and that if he had any money he should buy a lottery ticket. The bullet had entered Ivan's body on an angle, struck his rib, gouged the rib all the way around his body, and was lying under the skin of his back. It never entered his heart. Ivan walked out of the hospital the same day with just a couple stitches in his back from a cut to remove the bullet.

Ivan moved out of the apartment, and moved back home, to live with his parents in a nice two-story home on a quiet street. This was a typical home configuration built in northeast Philadelphia with a first floor entry garage in the front below grade with the living area built directly above it, and the bedrooms on the next floor. In order to enter the home, you walked up a walkway and climbed about four feet of stairs and entered to the side of the house over the garage. Late one night, several months later, Ivan came home and parked his car in the garage, but never exited the car. He fell asleep in the driver's seat with the garage door closed, and the motor running. It was in the newspaper two days later that Ivan and both his parents died that night from carbon monoxide poisoning.

PINNED

Our efforts were proving to be unsuccessful, probably due to the delay in starting effective CPR.

Ron and I received a call to go to the Reading Railroad terminal on Market Street to intercept a train that was coming in from the suburbs with a cardiac arrest patient on board. Evidently, the cardiac arrest happened when the train was a short distance from the station, so we were alerted to meet the train. Upon arrival at the station we were directed to the appropriate train platform a few minutes after the train had pulled in. About the fourth car down we found the door open, and the patient lying on the floor with several people in attendance. It seemed that no one on board the train knew how to do CPR so we had to work with what we had. We removed the patient quickly to the platform and began a short round of CPR and ventilation with oxygen before hooking the patient up to the heart monitor. The patient was a man in his middle fifties and appeared dressed for work. After looking at the heart monitor we noticed a fine fibrillation, and decided to try to get it coarse enough to shock. We started an IV and administered some epinephrine according to our proto-col, which did have a small effect on the heart but still not enough to shock. We continued to follow the protocol and administered more medication and eventually attempted the shock even though we were reasonably sure that the rhythm would not convert. Our efforts were proving to be unsuccessful probably due to the delay in starting effective CPR. We decided that we could do no more where we were situated, so the patient was made ready for transport to the hospital. In order to move the patient onto the stretcher and secure the equipment it involves a lot of moving around and organizing before the patient is lifted, and placed on the stretcher. When we finally picked the patient up to put him on the stretcher with the equipment, I noticed that I could not straighten my one leg, and my pants leg was part way up my leg and pinned to my knee. Upon closer examination I discovered that the angiocath we had used to insert the IV had impaled my pant leg to my knee. Further examination revealed that the dirty needle was driven all the way into the hub, effectively preventing me from straightening my leg. I grabbed the needle by its hub, and removed it, which allowed my pants leg to drop down to its normal position, and also allowed me to move my knee and walk on my leg. We never put any dirty equipment back in the drug box where it could contaminate all of our supplies. Any used disposable equipment was discarded at the scene, and in this case while moving around the patient working, I had knelt on the dirty angiocath. Since I was not sure of the cause of death of the patient, or any latent diseases he possessed I could not be sure what the future ramifications of this accident would be. Several months later I was to come down with a horrible case of lymphoma which resulted in the end of my fire department career. I always wondered if this incident contributed to the cause of my illness. It's something for which I will never receive an answer.

MMMMMMMMMM GOOD

Ipecac syrup is a solution, once swallowed, causes the patient to vomit. It's very upsetting to the stomach.

It was about 10 o'clock at night and we had to respond about 18 blocks to a home just off Center City. The radio gave us no information as to the source of the call, and what we were to encounter there. An older woman met us as the door and directed us to the living room of the home. Sitting in the living room was a younger woman who had taken an unknown quantity of pills in what was reported to us as a suicide attempt. The older woman produced an empty vial, which according to her was the medication the younger woman had taken. In cases such as this the treatment is guided by the Poison Information Center which is accessed by telephone. The Poison Information Center telephone number was posted inside the lid of our drug box, so we requested a telephone to make the call. The older lady directed us to a phone in the next room and I contacted a physician at the center. I read him the prescription from the vial and was directed to give the patient one container of ipecac syrup followed by a large glass of warm water. Ipecac syrup is a solution, once swallowed, causes the person to vomit. It's very upsetting to the stomach. The syrup is contained in a small, single-use cup with a peel back lid, so I gave the young lady one to drink. She picked up the container and swallowed the contents, and began to lick the inside of the cup to make sure she got everything that was contained there. She seemed to enjoy it immensely. Having never sampled the medication myself, I asked her to tell me what it tasted like. She launched into this very descriptive seminar on the qualities of ipecac, which she reportedly enjoyed very much. At that time the older woman produced a warm glass of water which the young lady drank, while we all stood by for the result. After a reasonable amount of time had passed the woman reported no nausea, so I called the Poison Information Center again and reported the result. He instructed me to open another container, and give her a second container of ipecac which was done. The older woman again produced a glass of warm water and this time carried in a bucket. As before, the younger woman licked the container clean, thoroughly enjoying the taste, and proceeded to sit back contented and drank her water Again, after a reasonable amount of time the young woman showed no sign of abdominal distress, and another call was placed to the Poison Information Center. The physician again informed me to give her a third dose of ipecac which emptied the drug box of that medication. Again the patient drank the ipecac with great relish, sat back, and polished off a third glass of water and informed us that she was reaching her limit, and did not think she could do another 16 ounce glass of water. At that point since we had no more ipecac on board, we removed her to the closest emergency room, where, upon leaving the squad she thanked us for the three tasty containers of ipecac. She marched on into the emergency room with her empty vial container, her mother, and a bucket, feeling just wonderful like she was out for an evening stroll. It was an odd case, not the same as many other suicide attempts I had seen. My thoughts went back to Annie Hayes, and a male hairdresser who had had an argument with his wife, and drank a bottle of hair bleach. In both of those instances the liquid consumed by the patient was fatal, and an attempted suicide became a suicide.

NO MOORE

I would run into her every morning in the break room
where she held court over a cup of coffee and a cigarette.

The fire department allowed firemen to work a side
job on their days off. Many firemen had their own busi-
nesses, and others worked for large companies like Sears
and Roebuck. I took a part-time job early in my career at
a mail order Sears plant where many fireman worked. It
was a very large building on Roosevelt Boulevard and it
employed hundreds of local people. I took a job there for
two reasons: the first was to meet girls, and there were lots
there; and the second was to afford new cars by subsidizing
my fire department salary. I worked on a floor that handled
catalog sales of infant and toddler items. There were a lot
of young black girls that would pick the items from their
bins and deliver them to a chute where they would be sent
to packing for mail order. Sitting at the chute was an older
woman who had spent a career working in that department,
and had advanced to the point where she was checking the
orders that were picked for errors. Her name was Gloria
Moore, and she was well known in the department for
speaking her mind. She had the best defense mechanism
of anyone I have ever run across, a big mouth and a quick
wit. I would run into her every morning in the break room
where she held court over a cup of coffee and a cigarette.

After several years of working at Sears, I moved on to
other side jobs, and I worked in a rescue squad that had
Sears Roebuck in its local area. One morning about 7:45
AM John Ondik and I received a call to respond to the
Sears Roebuck employee parking lot. It was a very, very

large parking lot with row after row of employee cars. After a few minutes we found the appropriate car surrounded by older women, all directing us to the rear seat. On the right rear of the car hanging out of the seat was an older black woman with her chin down on her chest, not breathing. We pulled her out of the car onto the ground, and began CPR on her immediately, although things looked bad. By our count, she had been approximately 15 minutes with no heartbeat or ventilation, so for the sake of all of the women present, we began to work on their friend. After some CPR she was connected to the monitor and as I suspected there was nothing but a flat line with no cardiac activity at all. We continued CPR as we began loading the lady onto the stretcher for transport to the hospital. It was then I had an opportunity to see her face, and I was sure it was Gloria Moore. I asked one of the ladies present if in fact it was Gloria Moore, and she said yes. It was the first and only time that I knew one of my patients. Gloria was pronounced dead at the hospital. I was sorry there was nothing we could do for her.

WHERE THERE IS SMOKE
THERE IS FIRE

*She had smoke residue all over her face,
but that could have come from her walking
around in a smoke filled apartment.*

One of the first things that you did when you came to work in the morning was to get a short report from the men you were relieving. If there were any cases during the prior shift, you wanted to do a physical check of supplies to make sure that you were equipped with everything you could possibly need on an emergency. You would also check to make sure that the equipment was spotless, and that everything was in its appropriate location on the squad.

We were in the middle of checking everything over when the call came in. It was reported as a possible fire in an apartment complex where neighbors smelled an odor of smoke in the first floor hallway and called in an alarm. Since we were already at the squad checking things, my partner had the jump on everyone else in the station, and we were out the door before the bells stopped ringing. The rescue being fast and nimble in morning traffic was the very first apparatus to arrive at the scene of the call. We knew that the call originated for a problem in the first floor hallway, so we made a beeline for that area. Surprisingly, there were no alarm bells going off, and all the apartment doors in that hallway were shut and secured. We felt like bloodhounds, sniffing the air trying to detect what had prompted the call. There was a faint odor of smoke that seemed to be in one area near an apartment door, so we knocked on that door first. In a few minutes after the second set of knocks the door cracked open when a woman in a house-coat answered. She looked rather odd, with what appeared to be goth type makeup, and moderate smoke drifted out of the small opening she was talking through. When we saw the smoke I pushed the door all the way open, and saw that the living room area was packed with smoke from the ceiling down to her chest. Both my partner and I rushed into the apartment and began searching the rooms for the fire. I went down the hall opening every door as I went looking for signs of a fire. By the time I reached the last bedroom my partner had found something in the kitchen, and called me back to that area.

What he had found was a frying pan in the sink with spilled cooked food under it, water all over the floor, and small burnt black pieces of cloth scattered around on the wet floor. The woman just stood there volunteering no information about what had transpired in the kitchen before our arrival. I began to question her about the mess in the kitchen, and when I looked at the meat in the sink I did not see anything that resembled burnt unattended food that was overcooked. She had smoke residue all over her face, but that could have been from her walking around in the closed smoke filled apartment. Eventually she said that she had a small cooking fire, but that she had put it out herself. But, I saw nothing to make the story believable. I bent down and picked up the biggest piece of burnt cloth on the wet floor and examined it. It was a white cotton fabric with a little blue flower on it, and immediately the bells went off in my head. I asked her to open her housecoat, and she refused. I asked her again, and in the distance I could hear a dozen men making their way through the building, the cavalry had arrived. The second time she opened her housecoat to reveal a naked horribly burnt body with pieces of cloth still burned into her flesh. She had been cooking in her pajamas over a gas stove and had caught fire. The fire was consuming her pajamas as she tried to secure the frying pan before attempting to douse her burning clothing. Eventually she was able to throw some water on herself, but someone on the way to work was alert enough to send in the alarm. She was in the bedroom when we knocked and threw on the housecoat to answer the door. She had no intention of either turning in the alarm or seeking first aid for her burns. We took her to the closest hospital, and she was later transferred to a burn center after her condition was stabilized. She never returned back to the apartment where her injury took place.

DEATH'S DOORSTEP

The Friday night shift was not very remarkable, except I had been experiencing a low grade fever with no rational explanation why. I was able to retire to the bunkroom about 2 o'clock in the morning when I experienced a pain in my upper leg at the groin level. I began to rub the area when I felt a small BB sized lump, which was the source of the discomfort. I roused my partner and headed for the closest emergency room to talk to a physician there. We went to Hahnemann Hospital where I was seen by the emergency room doctor. She examined me, but could not determine what was wrong with me. She gave me a prescription for a medicine called Keflex, and told me that if I was no better on Monday I should see my family doctor. I never made it to Monday, as I was so ill that I went to my local hospital on Sunday night and was admitted with a ping pong ball sized tumor in my groin and a high grade fever.

The tumor was removed in surgery, and the cell type was a lymphatic cancer which was very aggressive, and would completely change my life. By the next weekend I was on death's doorstep. Several cancer doctors were summoned on Sunday night and administered an experimental dose of chemotherapy with my wife's understanding that I may not survive the treatment long enough for it to take effect.

After two weeks of unbelievable suffering, I was discharged from the hospital and sent home to die.

I had lost over 30 pounds and was unable to eat from side effects of the chemotherapy. I was told to make an appointment with an oncologist for another dose of chemotherapy if I survived the three weeks until the dose was due.

During my time at home, firemen and officers were constant visitors to my home asking my wife if there was anything she needed, or if there was anything they could do for her. They offered pizza, steak sandwiches, almost anything that a fireman might like to consume. They offered to sit by me while she shopped, run errands, anything that they could do to make her life easier.

I went on for six months more suspended between living and dying, Every wound on my body became infected, old IV sites oozed puss. My wife fed me milk shakes with raw eggs, and other supplements in them in an attempt to help me gain weight. I would sit at the dinner table and cry because I couldn't swallow hot or warm food even if it was put in a blender.

Eventually I received another dose of chemotherapy, and vomited for 21 days around the clock, finding that both coke, and iced tea came back up better than green bile. With every visit to the oncologist's office I saw fewer and fewer of the patients I had talked to there. They all died one by one.

After over six months of chemo I was to receive a full body dose of radiation daily for eight weeks.

I had unbelievably gained back enough weight to take public transportation to the hospital where my radiation was to be given. On my first treatment I recognized a man who had undergone chemo with me. He was a wreck. He got his radiation just before me, and we talked every day while waiting to be called. Halfway through the treatments he died, and I cried all the way home, and all that night. I resolved that the cancer was not going to get me.

Eventually, the radiation was completed and unknown to me my skin would blister from the burning that the radiation had done. My intestines were also damaged; I had persistent diarrhea until they healed and could do their job again. I was on a plane going on a small vaca-tion to celebrate the end of my treatment when I became uncomfortable. I had a burning sensation all over, and when I undressed at the hotel I found that I was covered by fluid filled blisters, and horribly reddened burned skin.

After months of recovery I returned to work in Rescue 7 to the astonishment of several of the men in that station who had been informed that I had died. I was to go on for a short time working as before, when one day I was carrying a patient down a flight of steps when I made a misstep and smashed the head of my femur, bleeding into the joint capsule. I was to go on to have a total hip replacement on that hip which had been destroyed by both the chemo and radiation so close together. A year later I smashed the other head of the femur, and had that replaced with a total hip joint. I was thirty-eight.

After both surgeries, I was offered a job in Fire Prevention talking to school kids, but I refused, and left the department to make my way in the world. It was a sad day when I gathered up all of my uniforms, coats, boots, and gear and took them to the local firehouse to give to the men there. My original helmet is in the collection of my cousin William Bankhead a retired fire captain still living in Philadelphia.

EPILOGUE

Later in life, long after my bout with cancer, I decided that I would like to live in Florida. Doing due diligence, I found that I would need to acquire a vocation that would enable me to get a job in my new locale. I found that nurses were in demand at the time, and I decided to try a few courses at the local community college in Philadelphia. I was able to complete all the prerequisite work and get accepted by Thomas Jefferson University in their Health Sciences School, attending the Nursing Program. I completed the program, and graduated with a BSN Degree. I moved to Florida several days after graduating, and took a position at Largo Medical Center awaiting my licensure exam in Tampa, Florida.

After passing the licensure exam, I worked in the nursing profession for 18 years, eventually retiring in 2010. At present I reside in a retirement community in Pinellas Park Florida, and write as a hobby.

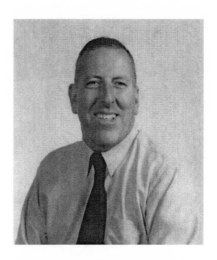

John Bankhead comes from a family of firefighters in the Philadelphia Fire Department. He was initially assigned to Engine 2 from the Fire Training School, at his father's request, to "get some experience". After an eight year career in both Engine 2 and Ladder 3, he moved into the old fire rescue service as it was expanding. After several years he was asked to join the first class of paramedics trained at Philadelphia General Hospital.

After completing his training and finishing second in the class, he was assigned to the first Mobile Intensive Care Rescue stationed in center city Philadelphia. After years of dedicated service he was stricken with lymphoma requiring double hip replacements, resulting in an end to his Fire Rescue Service. He went on to enroll and graduate from Thomas Jefferson University with a Bachelor of Science degree in nursing, and obtained his RN in the State of Florida where he now resides. He completed 18 years of practice in nursing, eventually teaching nursing for the last two years of his career.